T0129147

# STRESS
## MAKES YOU
# FAT,
# WRINKLED
## AND
# DEAD

*How To Avoid It!*

## BY PROF. ELIEZER BEN-JOSEPH
## &
## RICHARD H. LEWIS, M.A.

authorHOUSE®

AuthorHouse™
1663 Liberty Drive
Bloomington, IN 47403
www.authorhouse.com
Phone: 1 (800) 839-8640

Published by AuthorHouse  07/26/2017

ISBN: 978-1-5246-9241-4 (sc)
ISBN: 978-1-5246-9242-1 (hc)
ISBN: 978-1-5246-9240-7 (e)

Library of Congress Control Number: 2017907913

## Testimonials

### *Comments by Chris (Comeswithclouds) White "Stress Makes You Fat, Wrinkled and Dead."*

Something transforming showed up for me while reading, *"Stress Makes You Fat, Wrinkled and Dead"* authored by my friend of five years Dr. Eliezer Ben-Joseph and author Richard H. Lewis. After reading the manuscript and before this book even makes it to your bookshelf, my life is changed! I realize Dr. Ben-Joseph meant this book for me, and you – now!

Travel down this worthy path to eliminate stress, already paved by Dr. Ben-Joseph's near death experience. He is perhaps the most fascinating, accomplished and caring man I have ever met. His light humor beams throughout these provocative 22 chapters. Richard's talents also shine through as he uses what he and Dr. Ben-Joseph have personally learned from PTSD. They offer a fountain of knowledge transforming our ability to live longer and fuller lives stress free. Reading their shared words is like walking barefoot in a grassy park with dear friends who understand stress, pain, sorrow and loss. They understand our vulnerabilities. These authors are gifting you a golden chalice to help save your very life.

Both authors make foundational sound arguments while offering free medical hints and product advice from your eyes to your calluses, from your ears to your moccasins. They help you break down stress into easy to understand language and offer methods to melt away stress. They provide medical insight into everything from food, skin and sex to emotions and three-minute techniques to deal with stress and face problems head on. They highlight good news, a grand map, and dangers of suppressing anger. They explain what vitamins to add and which to remove, prevention by neoprene and solutions using bio-chemical research.

Honestly, this book surprised me by revealing my own struggles with stress. In my job with the Native American Church of Virginia, I am viewed as a spiritual leader and counselor. It is my job to encourage people who are suffering in this world of chaos, confusion and lies, in this interim reality of agreement.

Before picking up the manuscript, I prayed and pondered in what manner I would receive Dr. Ben-Joseph's request to write this forward, read this manuscript and rise to create space for the message and wisdom these authors are imparting in these 200-plus pages.

Immediately, the first sentence stopped me in the busyness of my head, "Stress…. Probably the very last thing you want to do when you are stressed is read a book…" Then Great Spirit whispered, "This book is for me and everyone now." … wow, this was just the first sentence.

As I began to read, my internal dialog debated and I countered with myself, "I have a handle on stress." "I am almost there." "I'll try this one more time." "Just a little longer." "One more project." "Then I won't have stress." Common excuses we all make, as if defending our own stress. But, not anymore! I was convicted. As a pastor and friend I realized I am not practicing what I preach. In fact, it occurs to me that I am a hypocrite. Ironic, as it may be, the time could not have been more right. "I am stressed out!" As I continued to read, I smiled and reflected a lot, "Wow. I am not alone, this book is for everyone."

I have never read a book, other than the Bible, that revealed as much truth and called me into such a profound state of personal conviction as this latest work on stress. I also believe we are loved so much that Creator is trying to speak to us through these two authors.

"*Stress Makes You Fat, Wrinkled and Dead*" also has references and parallels to my Native American Indian beliefs and teachings that we hold true. In the Native American medicine wheel of spring, summer, winter and fall, we are living and moving through different cycles, seasons and emotions as *'two-leggeds'* on Mother Earth. None of our paths are easy. But, if you think stress is a natural product of your life and nature's way, prepare to be surprised. Find the missing key ingredients to remove stress right here.

This book makes a case for all the areas of where stress gets a foothold in your life. This book is a treasure that shows how easy it is to get rid of: fatigue, headaches, depression, indigestion, anorexia, bulimia, and just about anything that comes from stress. Stress does not have to kill. Learn something you, "don't know, you don't know" to move on and get rid of stuff. Learn how to unravel the mystery behind the four types of stress. The authors creatively weave thousands of relevant questions helping the reader reach your own conclusions about yourself.

*"Stress Makes You Fat, Wrinkled and Dead"* is a solution to eliminate stress to create space, to be objective and present to what is real, what is true, what is really important, and to just be. In fact, read this book and "bounce" into a new way of being. Life is too short not to walk in more radiant, happier, healthier tranquility.

Get yourself back. Choose to live stress-free. Learn to plant seed and grow something good within yourself and for all your relations stress free. You impact the next seven generations. Let this book guide you now. Creator is calling. It is your choice. Create something good by your every step, stress-free.

If you or anyone you know is stressed, gift this book to them right away. Relief is a possibility you can create. I am sure that your reading this book will have profound and individual insights for you and the people around you.

For me the message I got was so simple, I would never have gotten it on my own. It has been right in front of my face the whole time. Stress is a choice. I have added this shocking revelation and natural recipe to my life, and my walk is already easier. After reading this book, I have made the choice that matters, to try to understand why I choose stress, and am learning to eliminate stress from my life while helping others reduce their own suffering.

Dr. Eliezer Ben-Joseph and Richard H. Lewis, I pray everyone is blessed by your literary collaboration and important contribution to help humanity heal.

**Chris (Comeswithclouds) White**
**CEO and Founder, Native American Church of Virginia Sanctuary**
**on the Trail**™
**www.SanctuaryontheTrail.org and www.HarvestGathering.org**
**ONACofVA@gmail.com**

**"Stress Makes You Fat, Wrinkled and Dead"Congratulations Dr. Eliezer Ben-Joseph and Richard Lewis, M.A.**

For the most part Stress is looked upon as being detrimental. Dr. Eliezer Ben-Joseph and Richard H. Lewis, M.A. have written this enlightening book of understanding Stress and finding solutions for the unavoidable stressors.

I see Stress as an *"opportunity"* to grow, to overcome adversity and a catalyst for peace and tranquility. Our happy receptors seem to be interfered with, when there is Stress or interferences.

Interference comes in on many levels. The Physical Body can experience Physical Stress through unseen radiations. As, in the case of electromagnetic influences coming from cell towers, computers, high frequencies – Gamma Rays & excessive air travel etc, which can harm the body. In addition, dangers from unseen chemical pollutions, which can cause the body to go into **Aniphilactic Shock and Adrenal Stress** as our natural response to poison. Our poor adrenal glands rise and fall to the occasion when we are stressed by these contaminants.

It is however, the mental and emotional radiations (stress) from people and relationships, whether it be family, friends, colleagues, clients or those that are in your field that can cause harm by Stressing your energetic fields through negative thought radiations (frequencies) towards you, or around you. Radiations can of course, also be supportive and loving, creating a positive influence.

What is stress? It is interference of the normal flow of life. There is but one life, One Energy that holds within a pattern of you connected to the universe. Your energy is part of the whole. We are part of earth. It is said; *when you move one grain of sand the entire universe feels it.* This illustrates how our environment affects us all. We find our friends and loved ones through the Great Law of Attraction.

The Universe consists of Positive and Negative Vibrations. When the two meet, a spark is created and a beginning can happen as energy begins to flow. When placing your hand on a patient to calm him down, or to boost his energy and give him strength… it is important to know the direction of this vital force. It is the Polarity of the electromagnetic field.

Stress affects the nervous system, and if it is out of balance, or in STRESS, the breath is the first key in knowing how to manage it. It is the air element that creates balance. Through the breath we can come back to our center and to the essence of our vital force! Within the breath there is an inhalation and an exhalation and it is between the breaths that the Aetheric Force Field resides. The Life Force (aetheric force) is a dynamic intelligence, which can repair itself, given the right environment. Good food, Good water, Good Air and Kind thoughts and Righteousness (right action). The body has an innate knowledge to heal. When stressed, it is our choice to make a change by actively sitting down to breathe, or meditate, or take a walk in nature and trust that the universe will support you.

Father Thomas Keating recently told me, that it is **in the "*intention*" of sitting in centered prayer that God/Peace/Divinity appears immediately!**

Stress is only a tool used by the higher forces to raise our own conscious awareness of who we are! Let us all deal with our Stressors and come to full awareness of why we are here. Our purpose is to expand consciousness from the plane of effects to include the plane of cause.

**Dr Linda Lancaster PhD, ND**
**Founder Global Foundation for Integrative Medicines**
**Founder Light Harmonics Institute**

## "Stress Makes You Fat, Wrinkled and Dead"
## Congratulations Dr. Eliezer Ben-Joseph and Richard Lewis, M.A.

One of the best things about this book is how Dr. Eliezer Ben-Joseph and Richard Lewis, M.A. explain basic, down to earth, how to deal with stress. Their coping strategies are sequential in nature and practical. For example, the authors give a step-by-step walk-through on how to engage a positive playground to share sexual pleasure, intimacy, trust and love.

The healing aspects are discussed as well with exercises for readers to engage in.

Because sexuality and love is important to many people as part of their personal belief system, I found Dr. Ben-Joseph's ability to offer insight into this topic impressive – particularly various aspects of a positive marriage. Some of the more concrete approaches to stress management are also discussed in the book.

Dr. Eliezer Ben-Joseph makes it a point in this book to approach wellness through the lens of mind and body, and dedicates an entire chapter – 10 tips for healthy eating. This is an area that many who write about stress often neglect. Because I have personally experienced the benefits of physical activity, walking or exercise related to mood, I was extremely glad to see that the author focused on chapter 7: "Walk off the pain" to this topic.

One of the things Dr. Eliezer Ben-Joseph and Richard Lewis, M.A. try to encourage clients to do is to think of wellness on multiple levels and not just the emotional or psychological. That's why they communicate the benefits of walking and health well!

### Final Thoughts

Stress is not always a bad thing. Stress is a reality of life, and believe it or not, that's not always a bad thing. It's amazing how much we can accomplish when the right amount of pressure is on. A manageable amount of stress by balancing the stress it can be extremely motivating. To prevent the accumulation of stress we need to resolve problems as they arise. Regular attention to the more relaxed side of life will actually increase your productivity because it relieves stress and leaves you feeling more resourceful. I encourage you to take a serious look at your life and take steps to lower, manage, and resolve the sources of stress you discover. Life is meant to be enjoyed... don't let anyone tell you otherwise.

This means learning to balance stress, so it doesn't consume us.

I have to say that I really enjoyed reading this book and will certainly use it for teaching and counseling purposes. It is also completely appropriate for anyone who is interested in living a healthier life.

The book, *Stress Makes You Fat, Wrinkled and Dead* by Dr. Eliezer Ben-Joseph and Richard Lewis, M.A. is one resource I will certainly recommend.

Thank you for reading, God Bless You.

**Rev. Minister Dr. Marwen Z. Saab N.M.D, Ph.D.**
**Knight of Grace of The Hospitaller Order of Saint Lazarus of Jerusalem**
**Prior of the Priory of Curaçao**
**Grand Chancellor General Magistral Council Sacred Medical Order of the Church of Hope**
**Papal Knight of his Eminence Pope Benedict XVI, Pontifical Order of St. Sylvester Pope and Martyr (Vatican)**
**CURAÇAO**

**Dr. Eliezer Ben- Joseph and Richard Lewis, M.A. Book**
**Stress Makes You Fat, Wrinkled and Dead**

When Dr. Eliezer Ben- Joseph, and Richard Lewis, M.A. first proposed the title and subject matter for their new book *"Stress Makes You Fat, Wrinkled and Dead,"* I was immediately reminded of the life work of my old friend and onetime mentor Dr. Lu from Denpasar, Bali Indonesia. Dr. Lu based his clinical practice in treating chronic and debilitating illnesses regardless of type or diagnosis on treating stress. He used to say Stress was the common and insidious cause, contributor and or exacerbate of all disease process.

I took this to heart.

I define a human being as a Stress Adaptive, Chemical-Biological, and Psych-Emotional, Transformational organism. We are from birth, adapted to living in a stressful environment. We adapt to stress and continue to remain adapting to our last day. Living is stressful and to be alive is to be subject to stress. This realization has figured prominently in the enlightenment process of many sacred sages and persons in virtually every religious philosophy such as in Buddhism's first noble truth. *"Birth is suffering; aging is suffering. Sickness is suffering; dissociation from the loved is suffering: not to get what one wants is suffering, in short the five categories affected by clinging are suffering."* [Samyutta Nikaya LVI, 11]

Stress is unavoidable. Therefore in and of itself, it is not good or bad. In fact, many kinds of stress – when handled appropriately and with positive adaptation and response to it – are stimulating to us. They help us to grow and to be better people. The idea is that if stress is the ocean we all swim in, than let's master this environment to the best of our abilities and learn to thrive in it.

Positive and conscious stress helps us to become well-rounded, mature and healthy balanced people. Unmanaged and or unhealthy stress (not handled or adapted to) becomes a force for deterioration and disease of every part of us – spirit, mind and body. So the trick is to become aware of the factor's inside and out, which form us one way or the other. Much research has gone into every aspect of this equation, and much research has been conducted; and much has been written on individual issues that are relevant. What Dr. Ben-Joseph and Richard Lewis, M.A. have done is to cut to the chase and in layman's terms, thoroughly covered the bases of the broad spectrum of sources of stress. And if not considered and responded to, or adapted to, will generate first: increasing dissatisfaction with life and eventually, contribute to ill health and a shorter and less productive life, which might have been possible.

Dealing well (or at least more consistently with stress), is so important, it definitely should top the list of those things for which we all should have been given a manual early in life… and mostly were not. *"Stress Makes You Fat, Wrinkled and Dead"* is that manual, a practical guide for moving into and living a healthier, happier and better-adapted long life. Therefore, the practical advise, abundant information, and the simple exercises will be of use to many.

**Prof. Anthony James DNM(C), ND(T), MD(AM), DOM, DPHC(h.c.), PhD(IM), PhD(h.c.HM), RAC, SMOKH**
**Dean, Professor, Director of Education and Traditional Medicine Chairman:**
**Oklevueha Native American Church of SomaVeda (ONACS)**
**SomaVeda College of Natural Medicine**
**The Thai Yoga Center**


**Stress Makes You Fat, Wrinkled and Dead**
**Dr. Zvenia**

It is my honor and pleasure to write this forward for Dr. Eliezer Ben-Joseph, as I have known this gentleman and friend/colleague for over thirty-plus years. Please note that Dr. Ben-Joseph is a respected naturopath and friend to many. It is with deep appreciation and his life long work to help others that has brought forward to fruition this new natural health masterpiece.

Please read and gain helpful insight to what natural health and all its components do with respect to general health and maintaining same. It is enlightening and a work to be treasured. I enjoyed this work and I hope you do too.

Sincerely,

*Benjamin Zvenia, NMD, MD (MA), Dr PH, JD*

## "Stress Makes You Fat, Wrinkled and Dead"
## Dr. Eliezer Ben- Joseph and Richard Lewis, M.A.

I love movies. I remember a funny line from a Steve Martin movie I once saw years ago, "Wow! Wow! Wow! All I can say is wow!" (Orion Pictures *Dirty Rotten Scoundrels* 1988.) However, being the practical man that I am, I would never dare to leave things at that; as clever and accurate though that Steve Martin line may be, particularly in this instance. I firmly believe in providing people with as much information as possible. Having as much available information as possible enables people to make fully informed decisions. That can sometimes be the difference between life and death itself.

I know stress; we are old foes. I've seen what it can do to people and have been so stressed myself that I honestly, for the life of me, could not even remember the make and model of my own car.

It is fascinating to me, even now, to ponder that thought but make no mistake; as fascinating as stress is, it has become common knowledge within the medical profession that it is also just as deadly. It kills slowly over time as it sneaks up on you while your back is turned from it.

In my brief lifetime I have been: an employee, a supervisor, a leader, a father, a husband, a student, a soldier, a police officer, a teacher, and many more things; all of which are stressful of course. I want anyone reading this and deciding whether or not to read this book that this book is for everyone and that it contains a comprehensive set of tools, techniques, and strategies designed to completely eliminate stress for those willing and able to read and heed.

Therefore, to quote another favorite line from another favorite movie, *"I guess it comes down to a simple choice really. Get busy living or get busy dying."* (Columbia Pictures *The Shawshank Redemption* 1994.) God bless: you, yours, the authors of this book, and our great country.

**Mike Nagle**
**Former El Paso Policeman,**
**Present English School Teacher**

## "Stress Makes You Fat, Wrinkled and Dead"
## Dr. Eliezer Ben- Joseph and Richard Lewis, M.A.

Prepare yourselves. Within these pages lie the secrets. What secrets you may ask? Well, in any good martial art school no one is taught the secrets right away. There is some time that must pass before a wise teacher can disseminate this invaluable knowledge to the student. In this way, the aspirant may achieve the proper state of mind necessary to continue the school's tradition. One must walk before one learns how to run. However, luckily for the reader, in this case, there is no need to wait. The secrets here are plain and simple. They are rational and straight-forward. They are the answers to life's age-old perturbations. Here is a book for *any* one of *any* age to learn what it means to live a happy stress free life.

Personally, I have only known Dr. Eliezer Ben-Joseph for a relatively short amount of time. As well, I too was only but a listener to his radio show. However, at the present moment I have had the unique and blessed opportunity to learn directly from the doctor himself. What led me here was my own personal journey into the realm of health sciences, which stems from my previous exploration of martial arts. Specifically, **Shaolin Chuan Fa, Tai Chi Chuan and Chi Gong**. And anyone who knows the doctor personally will tell you how much he loves martial arts. What does martial arts have to do with stress or health sciences? So much is the answer that a whole other book can be written on the subject. Here, though, we are talking about *"Stress Makes You Fat, Wrinkled and Dead."* The title alone will bring a smile to anyone's face, and believe me smiles are NOT scarce there at the clinic, as any one of his patients can tell you. In fact, it is rare to see a sullen face after a visit with Dr. Ben-Joseph. And when there is one, I can assure you, they must have the sensibility and sense of humor of a rock.

I would like to encourage the reader, you, to take some time out of your busy schedule to read this rare collection of quotable literature. Together, with the help of Richard Lewis, M.A., both he and Dr. Eliezer Ben-Joseph were able to compile a unique display of insight from the mind of the doctor; which is like an encyclopedia of information, especially in regards to health sciences. Along the way you will read the truths and you will find the secrets to dismantle any stressful situation. It's almost as if you are in the room with Dr. Ben-Joseph and he is speaking directly to you. I am positive that after putting this book down there will be a smile upon your face. For the one who has learned the secrets will surely be happy and stress free.

## Adan A. Baca
**Tien Shan Tzi, "Celestial Mountain Temple" Of Authentic Chinese Martial Arts**

# Contents

NOTES FROM THE AUTHORS.................................................15

CHAPTER 1:  STRESS .......................................................19

CHAPTER 2:  HARVESTING FROM THE SEASONS OF
LIFE ...........................................................31

CHAPTER 3:  NATURAL SOLUTIONS RADIO SHOW
QUESTIONS AND ANSWERS SAMPLE........43

CHAPTER 4:  MOVING ON .................................................53

CHAPTER 5:  FOUR TYPES OF STRESS .............................59

CHAPTER 6:  FROM THE GROUND UP STRESS CAN
MELT AWAY ..............................................69

CHAPTER 7:  WALK OFF THE PAIN .................................85

CHAPTER 8:  HELPFUL HINTS .........................................93

CHAPTER 9:  THE SOUND OF SILENCE............................95

CHAPTER 10: THE EYES ARE OUR GATEWAYS TO
HAPPINESS ............................................. 107

CHAPTER 11: SPEAK NO EVIL ........................................ 119

CHAPTER 12: WAYS TO DEAL WITH STRESS ................... 125

CHAPTER 13: WATER IS NATURE'S QUINTESSENTIAL
ANSWER.................................................. 129

CHAPTER 14: WE HAVE SEEN ENOUGH ......................... 135

CHAPTER 15: 10 TIPS FOR HEALTHY EATING ................ 139

CHAPTER 16: FOOD FOR THOUGHT GUIDELINES ....... 145

CHAPTER 17: LIVING IN OUR OWN SKIN ........................ 155

CHAPTER 18: CYCLES OF EMOTION................................ 167

CHAPTER 19: 2-3 MINUTE TECHNIQUES TO DEAL WITH
STRESS ................................................... 179

CHAPTER 20: SEX & RELATIONSHIPS.............................. 189

CHAPTER 21: ONE DEEP BREATH ....................................213

# NOTES FROM THE AUTHORS

## *Richard's Inspiration*

In the 1970s, I was trained in Manual Physical Therapy by Dr. Eliezer Ben-Joseph. This revolutionized my ability to help people who were in physical pain.

I always kept in touch with Dr. Ben-Joseph as both a mentor and as a friend. A few years back I was stressed out dealing with Life-long depression and Post-traumatic stress disorder (PTSD).

I was wrangling with inner demons that often come from PTSD and beyond.

One day a burning question popped into my head and I immediately called Dr. Ben-Joseph searching for my answer. He graciously talked me through my answers and solutions and the ease in which he shares information had us chatting for over an hour. Finally I said, "Well, I can turn this tape recorder off now."

He was thrilled to hear that I had recorded all his information and he said, *"I've only spoken in that detail to my mother."* Then he asked me to please transcribe it so that he could preserve the knowledge he had explained to me. That began a long series of conversations that we shared over many different topics and years.

Eventually we worked together for months on a radio script about stress entitled, *"The 6 Ways Stress Can Kill You."* When we were done, we performed the scripted interview and received accolades from the listening audience.

This led us to the idea of writing a comprehensive, entertaining and informative book on stress for you!

Of course, this huge task took years. In addition to our comprehensive book, you can find more stress tips and information on our website, where we show a rotating array of valuable advice and articles about stress.

Furthermore, tune in to Dr. Ben-Joseph's weekly radio show for additional information and inspiration.

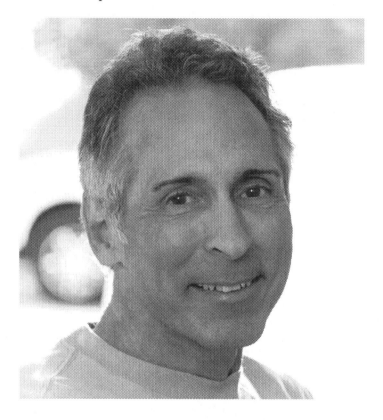

It is our wish that this book will give you the practical ways to free yourself from stress and provide the tools and the techniques to deal with any bumps in the road, remove roadblocks and barriers, deepen your intimacy and relationships; and add years to your lifetime.

Just the act of listening and learning, recording and sharing has changed my life immeasurably. I can tell you first hand this information really works. I am a living testimonial that one can be Stress-Free.

As we offer this incredible fountain of knowledge to all of you, I sincerely hope that this book will transform your lives beyond your greatest expectations.

Richard Lewis, M.A.

### *Eliezer's Journey of the Heart*

**Health** issues are running rampant in today's world. I have spent my life caring about the health of others. I believe the body, mind, spirit and soul can be healthy. We were born and designed to live an optimal and a healthy life. I have been recognized across the world as a Naturopath and a Healer. Yet, my satisfaction comes from sharing my knowledge, wisdom and understanding with you.

I have studied Natural Pure Science and Medicine. I have dedicated and spent my life researching the body – its systems, and the causes and reasons for illness, regeneration and pain. Today I have learned how to keep my kids healthy, my grandchildren healthy, my patients healthy and the world outside. There really isn't an illness that hasn't started from somewhere and that somewhere can be: tracked, unraveled, diagnosed and cured with proper understanding, attention, and the right avenue of healthy living and success.

I have taught doctors and therapists across the board and I have spent my weekends on the radio for years, helping callers live a healthier and a happier life and honestly so many of those calls are simply rooted from stress and I knew that this information could also help you.

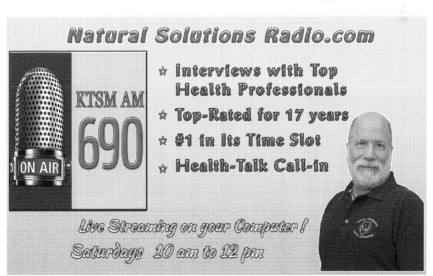

We started to write this book like a medical journal full of statistics and facts. Although they were all true, what we wanted most of all was to really assist you. So we've opened the pathways and the doorways to: your success, your journey, and happiness by guiding you to form your interpretation of your health, wealth, satisfaction, glory and ultimate wellness forever.

We are on the other side of the door; and are accessible to you every step of the way. We care in all earnestness about you, your wellness and your success.

This book offers the true keys, tools and secrets to a healthier and a happier life.

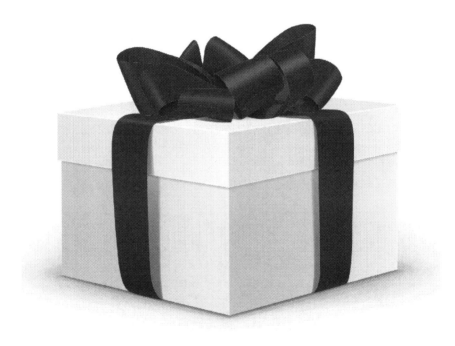

Find the section that pertains to you. Eat it up, devour the information, marinate in its truth and let it take you where you only dreamt you might live. Then we ask you to pass the book on, for another section may be just what your: friend, family member, loved one, colleague, or spouse may be yearning for. This book is the gift. Unwrap it with care, or go crazy and tear it apart like a kid on Christmas morning. Either way it is here, waiting for you.

# CHAPTER 1
# STRESS

Stress…

Probably the very last thing you want to do when you are stressed is read a book…

Wouldn't you rather: Scream, Yell, Throw Things, or Punch a Wall?

Maybe you'd rather: Run Away, Act Out, have Crazy, Wild Sex; or Eat All the Food in your Fridge.

What if that one book could change your life? What if even one page could offer you the tools, secrets or the key to an astonishingly happy and carefree life?

Then you would read it right? Lucky for you this book is in your hands! You are already half way there!!

First let's look at Stress: is it your boss, your job, your spouse, financial strain, a health issue or are you just plain having a very bad day?

We love the line from "Crimes of the Heart" when the police ask the main character why she shot her husband she replies, *"I was having a bad day… it was a very bad day!"*

The line always makes us laugh — obviously we are not going to kill our perpetrators; yet, we can kill Stress.

We've sectioned this book up into easy, fun, informative and eye opening pages. So if you don't have a two-year old that is running like a maniac thru the aisles of Toys 'R Us, you can turn to the page that's written just for you. That's right! We know what is going on in your life. We're kind of like a Santa Claus. We can see the good and the bad; and we can bring you a gift that can change your life. Today, Tomorrow and Forever… Yes!!! You can be, Stress Free!!

Our lives have been an action adventure movie, some people run from virtual tigers and demons. We've lived a life of amazing stories, scenarios, changes and events. And we've made it our life's passion to take all that knowledge and wisdom and to share it – with you.

Many people laughed at our title… **"Stress makes you Fat, Wrinkled and Dead"** — only guess what? It does! We have lived a life of wonder and excitement; and we have faced death, square between the eyes. We've traveled the world and we've learned a lot along our pathway to the human experience and healthy living. We've picked up enough breadcrumbs along the way to know that *"Fat, Wrinkled and Dead"* lives on the road and the pathway to Stress. There are other roads. So many beautiful ways to live this life and to enjoy this journey, we spent years slaying dragons and like David, the lessons were too great not to share. We realized as a doctor, and as an educator, that we could write the ultimate book that contains all the secrets and the pathway to Wellness, Health and Stress-Free Living. Periodically you'll find that we'll open the window to our own journey. This vulnerability allows us to uncover truths that have never been shared in a book before.

To learn how to: face and vanquish death, stay fit and trim, live joyously, and how to slay your own dragons, Read on…

There is a wealth of jewels waiting for you in these pages.

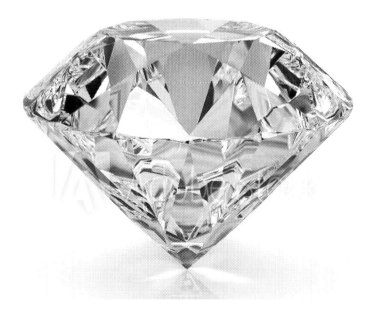

## The Stress Epidemic

Did you know that studies show elevated levels of stress in over 1/3 of Americans? We live in a free country and we're told we can be and do whatever we dream, and still we are stressed. Not only stressed, our relationships are deteriorating, our divorce rates are through the roof and our work productivity has dropped to drastic rates. That's insane!

We're told the leading two causes of this wide-spread epidemic are **Financial Stress and Job Stress,** creating stress levels that are rising off the charts. Remember when our ancestors came over on a boat (with people were dying around them)? They forged new roads and new avenues of living, with only pennies in their pocket, while carrying just their hopes and dreams. And today, we are **more stressed** – can that be true?

Looking at our news and community papers, we learn that it's commonplace to fight with those around us, even if it is family members and people that we love.

We've seen the increasing emphasis in the medical world has changed its focus to the whole person. That means your emotions are linked to your illnesses; and today, rapid deadly diseases are killing our spirits along with our bodies, and our future like never before.

Studies as far back as 1950 conducted by acclaimed researcher Thomas Holmes, suggested that people undergoing stressful situations such as: divorce, death of a spouse, or loss of a job, were more likely to develop tuberculosis, and less likely to recover from it, than those leading and living a stress-free life. The study showed the direct correlation between the culmination of hardship, and emotional havoc, and how it directly affects our health and wellbeing.

Recent studies from advanced immunology, and bio-statistics, suggest that stress may lead to decreased immune function and what we've come to know as clinical disease (diseases that are identifiable by chemical, hematological bio-physical, microbiological or immunological means: e.g. **air-borne disease, functional disease, immune complex disease, etc.**).

### Could this be you?

Do you know that studies show:

> ➢ 47% of people report lying awake at night

Are you tossing and turning? Walking your hallways? Jumping on your computer? Taking meds to fall asleep? Is this you?

> ➢ 43% report irritability or anger

Have you snapped at: your children, your spouse, your employees, co-workers, or even the waiter or waitress, or salesclerk? Have you found yourself short-tempered, grumpy, or downright mean sometimes?

> ➢ 43% report fatigue

Ah… this is a big one. How many times have you felt like: you haven't had enough sleep, or that you were too tired to work out, or have sex, or be motivated to start a new project, or even a new day?

> ➢ 40% report lack of enthusiasm: Are the sidewalks in your neighborhood cracked or uneven, has your car dipped into potholes, have they taken away the grass in your child's school, or are you eating fast or processed food all because it's easy, and just there. If you haven't stepped up in your life to make a difference, or to make a change for the better, this may be you!

> ➢ 34% report headaches. This is so prevalent in today's world. If you look at commercials on television from the 50's 60's 70's 80's 90's etc, it is rare to find a commercial for a headache. Now we have multiple products to stop the pain wracking our brain, and our mind from thoughts that are caused, you bet, by stress.

> ➢ 34% report feeling sad or depressed — even our kids today have a melancholy and sadness. The teen rate for suicide is at a frightening high. And bullying, peer pressure and just disconnection from others – whether by computers, or electronic

devises that split families, or the fast-paced society of today is tearing our kids and adults apart.

Loss of a job, money, a child, or an illness can cause a wave of sweeping sadness that some people never recover from.

> 32% report feeling as if they could cry, but why don't they? What holds back our emotions and our hearts? Is it our emotional shutdown, or a disconnecting from others, or our society's ever-increasing depression?

> 27% report upset stomach or indigestion. I actually think this should be a much higher statistic from: Acid Reflux, Crohn's Disease, Lactose Intolerance, Glutton allergies, and on and on. Not to mention the **emotional distress that our stomachs take as the brunt of our unhappiness, failures, pain, sadness or duress.**

From over-eating obesity or under-eating anorexia, bulimia, or just plain commercial fast food, our digestive tracts are on a rollercoaster of emotional chaos and stress.

This book covers the gamut of the whys — the problems and the solutions to the growing and widespread stress epidemic today. We're sharing with you the best and most effective tools to overcome any type of stress. May this book be your guide and your own personal roadmap to wellness, health, freedom and emotional, success.

**To Your Health and Happiness,**
**Dr. Eliezer Ben-Joseph**
**Richard Lewis, M.A.**

Stress... what does it mean? If you were little and you had trouble with your S's, and you've hated this word since you were small yet, what does the dictionary say Stress is?

1. Stress is a Noun... so is a chair, or a table, or whipped cream. **Stress is something we create.**

The dictionary says that it is **mental, emotional or physical strain, tension, or discomfort resulting from adverse conditions or very demanding situations.**

Does that mean: a snow storm, slick city streets, bearing a child, opening a jar, taking a test, raising our hands to answer a question, or saving a life is stressful? Is every firefighter stressed? Every boxer? Every pilot? No! Of course not! We don't all live in the pool of stress. So when does it happen and how can we eliminate it from our lives?

This book will unravel the mystery and shed light on the truth of the evil we've come to know as **Stressful Living**.

Did you know that statistics show that 47% of people report lying awake at night? Of course, those "people" referred to in this book, are not scared by Lions and Tigers; it's all about "You."

When you were little, you would lie awake thinking there were monsters under the bed or in the closet. As adults we still have our monsters and demons, only now they are in our life and in our head.

If you flip and turn to: watch TV, read a book, play solitaire or video poker on your computer, or wake up generally exhausted, or irritable – jump immediately to page xyz. If you sleep like a baby and wake up crying or hungry, or need to relive yourself, or wake up in the middle of the night just wanting love; then page xyz is for you.

For the rest of you who are sure you are just looking for the answers this book is your "Golden Chalice" and can change and save your life.

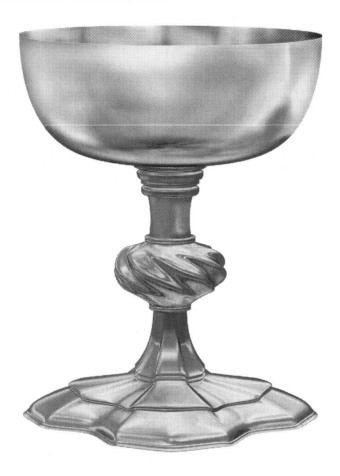

First let's start with one of today's leading cause of Financial Stress: **"Identity Theft"**

One woman who we know had her identity stolen, and her Mother said gently, "Honey you should take it as a compliment, that someone wanted to 'Be' you."

As sweet as that sounds, her life was turned upside down in turmoil: her accounts were emptied, her credit was damaged, and she was called into court for traffic violations that were in her name, while she wasn't even in town during the time of the problem.

How many people today have had their identity tapped into or their computers hacked? How many commercials advertise products, companies or programs to protect or to clean up your credit, or identity problems? Just reading about it makes one completely stressed out. So what can you do?

Immediately we are frightened and our bodies freeze, almost immobile; or we run as fast as possible to escape our fear. If you were running from a hungry lion, that would make sense. However, because someone has your Bloomingdales account number, your life is not in danger. First breathe; next make a plan of who do you call: the card companies, the credit bureaus, or credit protection agencies? **Help is available**. Unfortunately this is a true dilemma of the modern technological world today.

Never give out your information on the phone, or on the computer — protect who you are. You are precious and strong. Don't let anyone steal: your life, your happiness, your freedom – or twirl you into a stressful ball of nerves. Take a class in yoga or tai chi: swim, exercise, take a walk outdoors, or even have a good cry to release the stress. Know that holding stress in, and feeling frustrated at the world, will not change the situation. However, it might change you, your health and your happiness. For hints and secrets to immediately relieve stress: from creditors, collectors, government agencies, and little surprises like identity theft, you can easily dive into our **chapter of 2-minute techniques for stress free living.**

Another leading cause of stress is **Financial**. Have you lost your job? Have you lost money in the stock market? Sent a kid to College, or just met the prettiest girl in town and want to sweep her off her feet?

**Financial Stress,** (especially in **divorce, loss of job, loss of income, or bankruptcy),** has been known to cause: **heart attacks, personal injuries, weight loss, or weight gain, or even death.** Remember how excited you were to put a penny in your piggy bank? That feeling of accumulation, saving, financial gain or growing our wealth can be freeing and make you feel alive. Is there somewhere you are growing right now? Are you adding to your dreams?

Let's talk for a minute about the downfall of financial stress – let's lift up your spirits and your life with easy solutions and ways to live a better and a much happier life.

Does talking about or thinking about money make your brain freeze? Migraines are a modern-day phenomenon. Do you think Moses stopped before picking up his staff and parting the Red Sea and said, *"Wait I can't do this today, I have a migraine?"* Or that Mother Teresa stopped helping the poor, because there wasn't enough money in her pocket to feed the towns she visited? No!

So how can you relive financial stress? The first step is time… that's right, good old Father Time. Every one of us was born with a life. A life represents time. We had time to teethe, time to roll over, and time to walk. We had time to learn and time to grow. And you too, our dear friends, were given the gift of time.

Are you watching TV? Reading your e-mails? Tinkering with your car? Or are you spinning your wheels with unnecessary chores, imagined worries, video games or mundane routines? As they say in *Moonstruck*, *"Snap out of it!"*

One of the Secrets to Success in any Millionaires arsenal is **time management**.

Did you know that a home-based business could take less than 4 hours a day? **Home-based businesses** not only boost your income, they also offer tax discounts and write offs in almost every area of your life.

Just leaving your soap out, or the dishwasher detergent can be a write-off. Food on: your flights, your vitamins, your travel, your car, your phone, and Internet cable can all be business expenses, when you create a business from your very own home. Imagine giving sample products to neighbors, family and friends. How much fun would that be?

You my friend, could even deduct 25% of your rent and for 5 entire years, you need only make an "attempt" at a home based business to be able to write off major and minor expenses in your life.

Then of course there's **the budget**. We know… budgets are like eating your vegetables, you know, they are good for you. Just sit down honestly; no one is looking. No budget God is deducting points if you draw on it, forget things, and then draw arrows when you remember them and ask yourself; how much does it cost me to live?

What are my monthly expenses, my yearly expenses, play expenses? And how about my emergency expenses like a tire blowing, or the dog or cat going to the vet, or a work injury, etc? See how much money you actually need to breathe easy and have a great, fabulous and stress-free life.

Now go to the end of the year and see where you traveled, what you bought: a new car, clothes, a flat screen TV, etc, and project your year. Okay, how much did you spend on your desired year? Did that match the budget on the crazy sheet in front of you? Even it out, so you know honestly how much do you need for your year, and from here let's plan how to get there. What don't you need? What apps don't you use in your phone? What clothes have you never worn? What restaurants could you have simply lived without? Just fill in what you really do want. Create a master plan to watch your dreams come true.

Another fabulous way to be financially stress free is to **hire an advisor**. A Certified Financial Planner, Accountant, Stockbroker or Bookkeeper can change your life. We can't possibly know everything!

As much as we'd love to rule the world there are **people that specialize** in everything: singing, composition, health, and fitness. Eye doctors do not know what knee doctors know, and divorce lawyers and trademark lawyers know entirely different facts to help their clients. You may be the brightest bulb in the room and still need someone that specializes in IRS resolution, estate planning, wills; etc. Don't be shy, get help and you will immediately feel the financial stress melt away!

A clock is on a wall; a watch is on your wrist. They both tell time... so does your phone these days. What device you use to manage your time is up to you, yet it is crucial in a Stress-Free World to **Master Time Management** and to make time your ally, your *compadre* and friend. At the end of every life people say; I wish I had more time. No one ever says, "I wish I watched one more episode of *Game of Thrones,* or could check my e-mails once more, or I wish I could play with my Xbox one more time." Use your time wisely and Financial Freedom is yours.

# CHAPTER 2

# HARVESTING FROM THE FROM THE SEASONS OF LIFE

We remember reading about Bamboo trees, and what we found to be most extraordinary is the fact that a bamboo seed actually takes years to break the ground. Yet once it sprouts, you can't kill it; they are virtually indestructible. If you cut it down, and it grows back taller and stronger than ever before. We always imagined the loving, patient person that every day watered the ground: knowing and trusting, that there was a seed just waiting under that earth, to one day burst through, and it would continue to flourish and grow.

***Be patient, plant your seeds and wait in joyful anticipation for the life you knew you could live.***

Many things in our lives have been the impetus for discovery and fortitude. So many treasures have passed our way, and so many memories still live within us. When we wrote this book, we sat and contemplated, asking ourselves the grand question – what were our greatest influences? We also wanted to share stories in which the framework of healing, health, wellness and the human heart could touch the world.

We remember watching the movie "Being There," a classic tale that is still a film favorite today. The story of 'Chauncey the Gardner,' played by Peter Sellers, drove us to share our knowledge in a deeply profound way.

Chauncey had never left the estate and all he knows of the outside world is what he has seen on television. When his benefactor dies, he is thrust out into the world. Hailed as a genius for his simplistic approach to life, he winds up by accident, in the game of politics. Then, through an odd series of circumstances, he becomes a personal advisor to the President of the United States. Chauncey has spent his entire life working as a gardener, and all he knows is how to tend the garden during the seasons. Chauncey's simple words about gardens and the weather are interpreted as allegorical statements about business and the state of the economy.

We wrote this article many years ago back in that time frame and it still holds true. There is a **Season for Everything** and now, it is "your" season for financial and spiritual success. It is the Season of growth, harmony and stress-free Living.

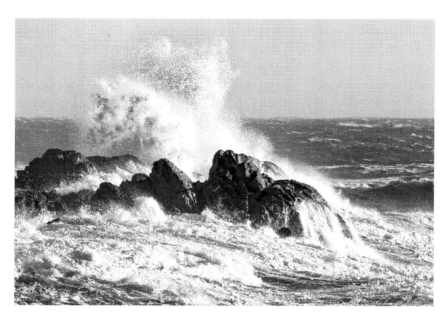

The tide comes in, and then recedes. The sun rises, giving light, and sets bringing darkness. Drought plagues the fields of the world, followed by heavy rain in abundance. The heat of the August sun gives way to the penetrating cold of the winter storm. The smile gives way to the tear.

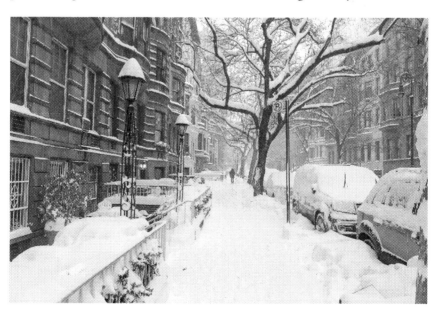

For each of us, existing on this blue-white sphere called earth, the wheel of life continues its constant turn. All human emotions appear, disappear, and appear once again. For all of us, the only constant factor in life is that we learn to experience the changing of life's cycles, without being changed by these cycles. To make a constant and conscious effort to improve ourselves in the face of changing circumstances, is to assure a tolerance for life's events; and to permit ourselves the full enjoyment of the blessings of life's harvest come the autumn.

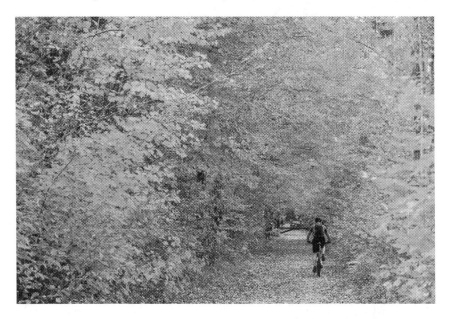

These then, are the cycles of life: the first, springtime, is the time to take advantage of opportunities, friendships, love and new ideas.

Springtime follows the turbulence of winter. It is the season of activity. It is the time to plant, and enter our fields of life with the seeds of knowledge; and a commitment of determined effort. Spring comes with its abundant beauty. Yet, do not be lulled into inactivity, soaking in the aroma of the fragrance of blossoming flowers. Otherwise, you will awaken to find planting season over, with your seed still in your sack.

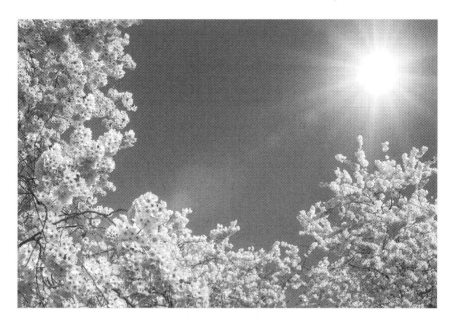

Remember the seasons come without emotion and care not what you do. **It is God who gives you the wisdom to know when to rise from your comfortable chair. And it is you, who must dig deep and find the discipline within yourself to make the effort of tilling and planting the fields.** Those fields are your mind and body, and it takes effort to keep them both healthy and strong.

The springtime of life does not come often. So do not let it pass you by, while you contemplate the hardships of the past winter of your life. Remember, if you want to know what tomorrow will bring, look at what you are doing today.

Given the gifts of intelligence, wisdom, and freedom of choice: as humans we are bestowed the discipline to plant in spite of the rocks, weeds, or any other obstacles before us.

To take full advantage of the spring, rid the soil in your mind of the weeds and rocks disguised as **negative opinions, worry, doubt or pessimism**. It is the fertilizer of **faith, love, enthusiasm**, and your efforts that will overcome the worst forms of bugs and weeds.

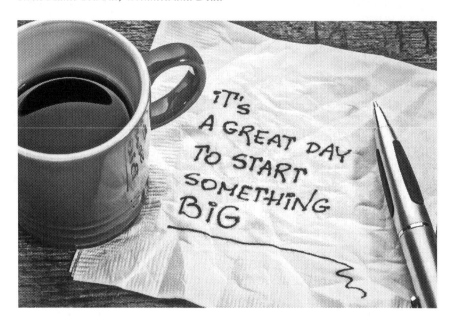

Springtime merely says, *"Here I am!"* So choose action, not rest. Choose truth, not lies. Choose a smile, not a frown. Choose love, not hate.

Life provides no assurance that the planting of seeds will provide the reaping of a harvest. Yet, to expend no effort during the spring will assure no results, come the fall.

Every seed produces its own kind: A seed of doubt, or fear, or distrust placed in the mind will also produce its own kind – inaction, pain, fatigue, or the inability to do your work. The price, or effort, of thinking thoughts of love: prosperity, or self-confidence is no greater effort in the mind than the price given to thoughts of hate, poverty, or self-doubt. Only the rewards are different. Each day is given to us as a new season of spring. The thoughts, deeds, dreams and efforts of will provide tomorrow's harvest. **There will be: no better day, no better opportunity, no better springtime, no better time to begin than the current moment. Seize the moments, as you find them, and mold them into your better future.**

**"Summertime is a time to protect and nurture."**

Success in life is not an easy matter. Nor is it an easy matter for the seed to push away the soil, in its quest to reach the light that brings it life and health. The spring is a time for the creation of things of value, and those things now require the season of summer for growing and gaining strength – that they might yield their harvest the coming fall. Develop an understanding and awareness of the fact that **good will always be attacked**. It is nature's way. Learn to accept the existence of negativity. Expect adversity for it shall surely appear. **Be grateful for adversity, for it forces the human spirit to grow. Human character is formed thru our response to difficulty — not in the absence of difficulty.**

All things, even adversity, have a worthy purpose. Let's face it... there will be people and events that are going to hurt you, and disappoint you. It has been this way through recorded history. Since you cannot control: the weather, or traffic, or your boss, or your neighbors, or the ones you love, then you must learn to control you — the one who's response to the difficulties of life really counts.

**Do not doubt yourself, for where doubt resides, confidence cannot. Do not neglect yourself in diet and exercise, for with neglect comes the loss of your health.** Do not imagine yourself to be less than you are, or more than you are. **Seek always to become all of which you are capable.** You are a fertile seed of the creator of all things, destined to live and not lie dormant, to spring forth from the soil called life, and grow upward toward the endless horizons of unlimited potential.

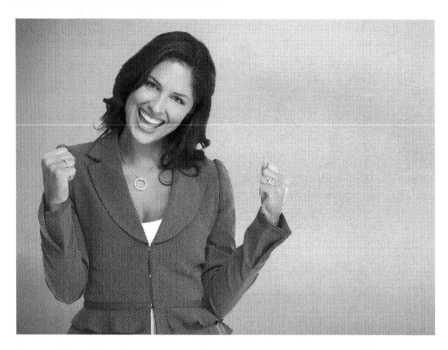

**It is your destiny to tap your talents, and to achieve all of which you believe yourself to be worthy.** The fall is a time for harvesting the fruits of our springtime and summertime labor. Fall is a time for rejoicing, as well as a time for a searching of the conscience.

For those who planted abundantly in the spring, and who fought against the bugs, weeds, heat and the weather of summer; fall can bring rewards of harvest. Nothing is more exciting than a full and wonderful crop, and nothing more dreadful than a barren field in the fall. So it is with those given the responsibility for planting, and so it is also to those who are given the responsibilities of life. An unproductive and meager harvest makes confession of our own past failures both difficult and necessary. The law is simple, and known to all. The law is **"As you sow, so shall you reap."**

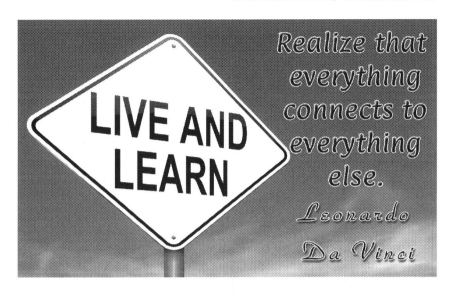

**In all areas of the human existence be aware that what we put into this world, we get back from it. It is the true manifestation of the law of cause and effect.**

In the fall, we either enjoy, or we excuse. **For those who failed to take advantage of the spring, and who failed to guard their crops throughout the heat of summer, there can only be excuses; and excuses are merely attempts to place the blame on our circumstances – rather than on ourselves.**

When you realize that your life is not about how you appear to others, **it's about how you feel about yourself.** And when you realize that your happiness is not about how much money you have in the bank, rather **it's making the most of what you have, and really enjoying those who are important to you**. And it's also how much effort you put into creating the life you desire. **In this way, you create your own happiness.**

**The key is to keep company only with people who uplift you, whose presence calls forth your best. – Epictetus**

**It's not what happens to you, but how you react to it that matters. – Epictetus**

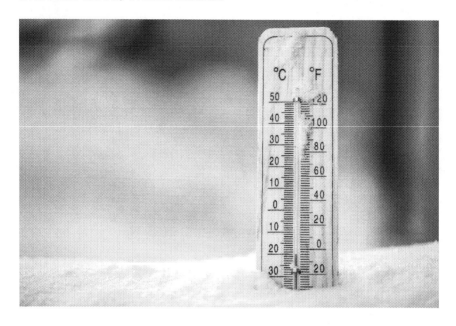

Winter — Prepared or Unprepared.

*A great lesson of life to learn is that winter will always come.*

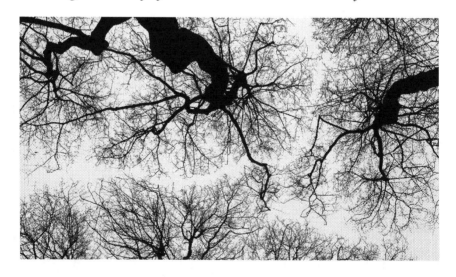

Not only the winter of cold and wind, and of ice or snow: but also the winters of despair and loneliness, or disappointment, or tragedy. **It is winter when we think our prayers go unanswered, or when the**

**acts of our children leave us shaken, or stunned.** Winter comes in many forms, and at any time, both to the planter of crops; and or to our personal lives.

The arrival of winter finds us in one of two categories: either we are prepared, or we are unprepared. To those who are prepared, who have planted in the spring, guarded their crops during the summer, and harvested during the fall, winter can be yet another season of opportunity. It can be reading for study, a time for planning, for gathering our strength for the coming spring. It can be a time of great enjoyment; a time to share with those we love. Winter is a time for rest and recuperation, a time to enjoy the fruits of our labors. To those who are unprepared, the arrival of winter is a time for regret and a time for sorrow.

Without the pain of earlier discipline, we pay the heavier pain of regret. Regret is an empty cupboard in your kitchen.

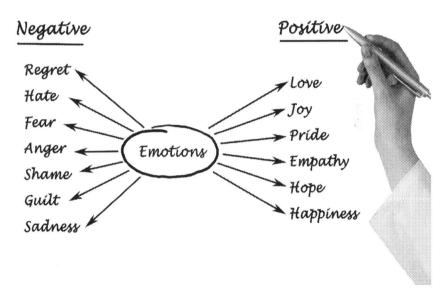

For things or circumstances to change, human attitudes, opinions, and habits, must also change. Let winter find you planning for the arrival of spring: with appreciation of the past, with gratitude for your achievements, adversities, and uncertainties of life. For each of these, is a blessing, which removes limitations from the possibilities of life.

Winter is a time for examining, pondering, and introspection. Winter is the time: for going within, and being sincere, with ourselves and about ourselves. Constant, gradual change is the order of the universe and only those worthy human attributes of: honesty, loyalty, love, and trust in our own abilities, and our God, are to remain constant.

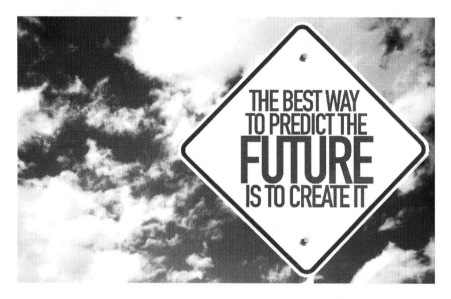

Winter is a time for being grateful for our achievements, or for having the strength to endure our lack of achievement. Don't pray for things to be easier, rather, **pray for more strength to handle obstacles and more challenges**, for it is out of these that man's character and will to succeed are formed.

# CHAPTER 3

# NATURAL SOLUTIONS RADIO SHOW QUESTIONS AND ANSWERS SAMPLE

**Question from Linda. Why are vitamin products, like B-complex, sold as Mg, while Vitamins E, A, and D sold as IU?**

B-vitamins and vitamin C are water soluble, which your body cannot store. Therefore, whatever amount you take in a day, the excess is flushed away in your urine. These substances are measured in milligrams (mg).

However, oil soluble vitamins as vitamin A, D, and E **are stored** in the body, and if one takes an excess of a proper dosage, that extra amount may build up and create telltale symptoms. These substances are measured in international units (iu).

**Washing Your Hands**

**Question from Alana**

**Every flu season I hear that doctors say the best way to protect yourself from the flu is by washing your hands regularly. However, they never really explain how we should wash our hands. Do you have any advise?**

Yes Alana, I'd be happy to describe what they mean. The proper way to is to wet both hands with clean, running water (warm or cold), and apply regular soap. Rub your hands together to produce a lather (a foam); while you scrub them well. Be thorough and wash the back of the hands, between the fingers and under the nails. For the nails, you can use a nailbrush for enhanced cleaning.

Keep washing for 20 seconds – the CDC recommends that you sing the "Happy Birthday" song two times. After this, rinse under running water; then dry the hands with a clean towel (**must be really clean** or else you are contaminating more bacteria to hands), or air dryer.

As an added protection I also rub 3 to 4 drops of a good essential oil into the palms of my hands (I use doTERRA essential oils as I think they are the best). I also rub the tips of my fingers on my palms, this way I put a protective barrier against any pathogen directly on my hands.

**Question from John. I have this running debate with my buddy. He says drinking orange juice is the same as eating an orange. I disagree – who's right?**

Well John, thanks for listening to the show. You are both right in different respects; let me explain. The general advice is to opt for the whole fruit because juices are stripped of the fiber, which most us don't get enough of. Also most juice contains a lot of sugar, which most of us consume too much of.

There was a study published in the *Journal of Agricultural and Food Chemistry* that was quite interesting. The study started with fresh navel oranges that were analyzed in three different forms: peeled segments, a mashed-up puree, and as juice. They also tested both fresh-squeezed and pasteurized juice. They found that levels of vitamin C and carotenoids were basically the same in the juice and the unprocessed fruit, while levels of flavonoids were significantly lower.

Then the scientists tested the oranges in a test tube model designed to mimic digestion, and what they found was very interesting. Much more of the carotenoids and flavonoids were released from the orange juice than from the fruit slices or mush. The differences were quite striking. The carotenoid release went up from nearly 11 percent in the fruit to 28 percent in the fresh juice, and up to 39.5 percent in the pasteurized juice. Meanwhile, flavonoids were boosted nearly five-fold in juice compared to fruit.

**Wendy White, a professor of food science and nutrition at Iowa State University, notes that drinking fruit juice spikes blood sugar levels more, and faster, than eating whole fruit. In addition, one Harvard study linked regular juice consumption to an increased risk of type2 diabetes. Those downsides of juice far outweigh any boost in carotenoids.**

Also, unless your bottle is sterilized glass, you also introduce other bacteria into the equation. Forget about plastic bottles! We know of the harmful effects of plastics in food packaging.

**Question from Maria. I have a weak immune system so I need to incorporate a powerful A-Z supplement to keep my health up.**

**Is there one you would recommend?**

Maria, I couldn't have asked for a better question. Let me tell you about the best A-Z anti-aging supplement, (that I personally designed and manufacture), called **Prime Longevity** – the most potent 6-tablet per day formula available anywhere.

The first question is how much of each nutrient do you want to consume? The amounts of each of the nutrients that are in **Prime Longevity** are the same amounts, or higher, that were in the scientific studies. These are real therapeutic amounts, not the miniscule amounts found on most supplements (just so that nutrient can be listed on the bottle, although they have no real benefits).

Also, the only way to get the higher amounts of these special nutrients – that you can't eat in foods, to produce the most potent formula – is with a 6-tablet product due to the sheer mass required to deliver such potency.

Secondly, there is no contest when you compare the nutrient amounts between **Prime Longevity** and any of its closest competitors. In addition, Prime Longevity contains a large amount of specialized nutrients that are very difficult to get in even the best of diets. Let me give you some examples:

**Resveratrol 120 mg:** is a natural compound that is found in: grape skins and seeds, pine needles, different berries, and of course red wine. Resveratrol is used **medicinally as antioxidant and anti-inflammatory,** and they may protect against cancer and cardiovascular disease. Resveratrol has also been shown to **slow down the aging process – and even reverse signs of aging!**

**Chromium polynicotinate 1,200 mcg:** is the only Chromium product that satisfies all of Dr. Mertz's laws to be established as a true **Glucose Tolerance Factor Chromium** (GTF); and **Chromium Polynicotinate** is the correct form. **Glucose Tolerance Factor Chromium is the form of Chromium used in all the research for improving weight loss and in controlling sugar metabolism, thus benefitting Type2 Diabetes.**

Chromium is a very important mineral, which works with vitamin B3 (niacin) in maintaining blood sugar levels. **Glucose Tolerance Factor Chromium** has recently been given a US Patent **because of this singular nutritional importance** – and also because of its **ability to lower cholesterol.** GTF Chromium is known to activate enzymes for carbohydrates, fat, and protein metabolism. **Chromium is also thought to aid the body in improving its circulation for healthy skin and hair.**

**CQ-10 120 mg: There are two forms of CQ-10: Ubiquinol and Ubiquinone, which both support cardiovascular, immune, and nervous systems, and promote longevity. Prime Longevity contains the stable form of Ubiquinone.** Don't fall for the advertising hype about Ubiquinol being more absorbable, **as all Ubiquinol turns to Ubiquinone in the stomach.**

**Selenium 240 mcg / Krebs cycle selenium:** Selenium is a natural trace mineral that works as an antioxidant, by scavenging cell-damaging **"free radicals." Prime Longevity** contains the **Krebs Cycle Selenium,** which has been studied for its greater effect on cancer. Selenium also benefits thyroid activity and is often used for weight reduction programs.

These are just some of the unique, super ingredients that make **Prime Longevity** the overwhelming champion of potency.

Now you're waiting to hear "… **and that's why this product costs so much – no way! Prime Longevity** has **top potency for less money!** It costs far less, and delivers more than you could ever do for yourself. It is the true meaning of getting 'Health Insurance.' (Prime Longevity's closest competitor is **triple the price!**)

**How the Thyroid Works**

This complex answer is long and complicated with a huge amount of medical knowledge. Therefore, it may be difficult to follow along, however, the answer is totally correct.

**Question from Shirley. Good morning Shirley, how are you?**

**Shirley** - I'm doing pretty good, thank you. Thank you also for being there, you do such great work.

**Dr. Ben-Joseph**

**I have a daughter who is going to the Doctor on Monday, and she thinks she has a thyroid problem, and I do too. I told her she needed**

**something beyond the TSH, but I don't remember what it was she was supposed to have exactly.**

Oh a good question and a question for everyone.

Patients complain to their doctors of common hypothyroid symptoms yet because their TSH falls in the 'normal' range, (0.5 to 5) their thyroid is declared normal. They are complaining of fatigue with insomnia, weight gain, loss of libido, muscle aches and pains all over, and depression. And their doctors will write them prescriptions for sleeping pills and anti-depressants, or pain medications, and tell them to just exercise more – implying that it's all in their head, instead of treating the underlying thyroid issue. We now only treat by the numbers and no longer treat the patient. How can doctors diagnose and treat thyroid disorders without doing a full investigation?

So what she wants is a complete thyroid profile. A full thyroid panel for hypothyroidism needs to include these 6 key thyroid lab tests: **TSH, Free T4, Free T3, Reverse T3, Thyroid Peroxidase Antibodies, and Thyroglobulin Antibodies.**

There is one major problem when you do thyroid tests; they only show circulating thyroid – and not cellular thyroid function. The problem with this approach is that thyroid physiology is complex. The production, conversion and uptake of thyroid hormone in the body involve several steps. A malfunction in any of these steps can cause hypothyroid symptoms. True cellular thyroid is tested by taking the body temperature.

Prepare the thermometer the night before, and take your body temperature first thing in the morning (before you stand up). Your normal temperature will read 97.8 or higher. Take your temperature again before dinner. Your normal temperature will read 98.4 or higher. When your body temperature is consistently below normal at either time, more than likely your thyroid is low, no matter what the blood chemistries are reading. **The body temperature is indicative of how thyroid is working on a cellular level,** not just the production of T4 in the thyroid gland.

Another major problem with thyroid testing is the role of Iodine. Look at the Periodic Table of Elements, column VIIB. This column is called the

Halogen group of metals, and the brain thinks they are all the same and interchangeable – they are not. In that column you're going to see a list of elements. The higher up the element occurs on the column, the stronger the element is. **Fluorine is at the top: then Chlorine, Bromine, Iodine, with Astatine at the bottom.** Astatine we don't care about, and it is at the bottom. Next up the list is Iodine, followed by bromine, chlorine, and fluorine. Let's look at how Iodine works in the body.

Iodine is a disinfectant; it kills things like bacteria and yeasts, and deactivates viruses. The blood circulates and makes a complete circuit around the body every 8 to 9 minutes. So that means the blood flows through the thyroid coming in contact with the thyroid hormone T4 every 8 to 9 minutes. The **T** is the amino acid **tyrosine,** and the **4** are found as the 4 atoms of iodine. So this means the blood is bathed in iodine and is disinfected continuously throughout our lives. When the rest of the body needs iodine, the pituitary secrets TSH (thyroid stimulating hormone), so the thyroid makes more T4 and sends it directly into the blood stream. Some of the T4 goes to the liver, some goes to the lung, then the kidneys; and lastly to the pancreas. The T4 drops off one of the iodine atom in those organs and goes back into the blood stream, (less one iodine atom), becoming T3.

Now the T3 is circulating in the blood stream and anything that comes in contact with the T3 is also disinfected. The T3 goes to the cells of the body and sticks to the surface of the cell and leaves one iodine atom on the surface of the cell and then goes inside the cell becoming T2. On the surface of the cell, the iodine disinfects anything that comes in contact with the cell. Inside the cell, one of the iodine molecules goes to the mitochondria (where energy is produced and also disinfects the mitochondria), losing another iodine molecule to become T1. The last iodine goes into the nucleus of the cell – now $T_0$ – and prevents any genetic mutations when the cells divide.

This is the roll of iodine in the body; it disinfects and keeps the body free of disease. So when the thyroid is healthy: and you have enough iodine for every cell in the body, you can't get a viral disease, or a bacterial disease, and you can't get cancer. Can this be the underlying reason that the thyroid is not treated properly? Can the poor treatment of thyroid really be withheld over money $$$?

Now let's go back to the periodic table of elements and see what happens to the iodine when there is not enough to overcome the laws of chemistry. How many people do you suppose eat something from a processed grain, and how often? Processed grains such as: bread, tortilla, pasta, noodle, cake, pie, cookie, muffin, chip, or any other processed grain product? The preservative in all of these grain products is **bromated vegetable oil,** in other words it is bromine. **Bromine sits above iodine so it is stronger and displaces the iodine off the T4 thyroid.**

Another question to ask is how many people still drink tap water or shower in tap water? The water contains chlorine, and it is above bromine on the periodic table. A 10-minute shower is the same as drinking 10 glasses of chlorinated water. As the chlorine is above bromine – therefore is stronger than bromine and iodine, **it continues to displace iodine off the thyroid.**

The last question is how many people use fluoride toothpaste to brush their teeth? **The last element at the top of the column is fluorine: and it is above chlorine, bromine, and iodine, and again is stronger than iodine and displaces more iodine off the thyroid hormone.**

So we go back to the thyroid blood tests and what happens is that the blood tests come back in the normal range. The TSH comes back normal or even low, and sometimes it might come back in the high range. Checking the free T4 or the free T3 may still come in the normal range, yet there is no iodine – so the thyroid can't work. **Remember these blood tests only reflect the circulation of the thyroid and not cellular iodine and true thyroid usage.** What I have described is normal laws of chemistry and is not mysterious. Have doctors, especially those that deal with thyroid disorders – the endocrinologists – somehow just forget chemistry?

Most of the U.S. population, no matter the age, is deficient in iodine; so people can then supplement with iodine. One of the most common forms of iodine is **Lugol's solution**. You build up slowly to about twenty-five to fifty milligrams of iodine, not micrograms. Lugol's Iodine is 6.25 mg. of total iodine. You start slowly with 1 drop per day in water or juice; and add 1 drop every 4$^{th}$ or 5$^{th}$ day until you reach 5 drops. Stay at that dose for about 1 year, as it takes about a year to flush the fluorine, chlorine, and bromine out of the body. Stop brushing your teeth with fluoride toothpaste, stop drinking chlorinated water and stop showers in tap water. Also stop eating regular processed grain, or any wheat bread products, because all of your bakery goods contain bromide (it is used as the preservative). So this is why your thyroid is not working. We tell people, 'do not use the blood test for your thyroid evaluation.' Because it doesn't always give you the information you need.

You may have a slow heart rate and low blood pressure; and maybe have yellow skin if you eat too much **beta carotene**. You can also get tiny bumps on the skin of the backs of your upper arms, or the back of the upper thighs. They almost scratch off like a little waxy stuff coming off under your fingernails.

Shirley, thank you for the question. I hope everybody gets a better idea of how the thyroid works. Remember go by the symptoms that your body is telling you. **Those of you that are suffering from fibromyalgia or chronic fatigue syndrome, they are one hundred percent low thyroid.** Every doctor in the world knew this before 1973 – it manifested as generalized muscle aches and pains with severe fatigue. So don't be short changed and let your doctor continue treating you with pain meds, anti-inflammatory meds, or anti-depressants. The real culprit is that your thyroid is still not working properly. Thank you again Shirley, there's our music and Dr. Eliezer Ben-Joseph will be right back with *Natural Solutions Radio*.

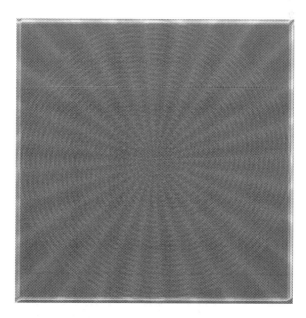

# CHAPTER 4

# MOVING ON

Okay, so it's the season and the time to move… *"Good Grief,"* says Charlie Brown. What could be more stressful than moving? Your life: your childhood, your memories, your family, and your precious possessions are all tucked into boxes and hauled away — it's crazy-making indeed. So whether your child is headed off to college, and you're about to enter the empty nest syndrome, or you just got transferred by your company to another state or country; **moving is one of the top causes of stress in the world today.** Buying a house, changing homes, packing away our lives: going thru our past, throwing away cherished memories and moments and learning *"who we are,"* happens naturally as we carefully box our worlds. And as we leave another chapter behind, the strain can often wreak havoc with our emotional systems, and with our lives.

Do you remember the first time you moved in with someone? Maybe it was: a brother or sister, a grandparent, a dorm room, a roommate, a lover, a spouse or even moving into assisted living, back with our children, hospice care, or to another war zone or space. Moving literally pulls the rug out from under our lives. Imagine being knocked over by a big wave and you've lost your footing, and then fear and panic set in. Moving knocks us about, and stress sneaks in thru the open door just begging for attention. And we're often too tired and too exhausted to close the door and lock it out, and send it on its way. So there it is a companion (among the tape, boxes and markers), just waiting to be carried from place to place.

Wouldn't it be wonderful to enjoy your future with eagerness and anticipation? Now that sounds like an exciting approach to your future and the fulfillment of your dreams.

**Where does one begin?**

The best way to reduce anxiety is not to think of the entire move at once. Instead, focus on each part separately. Boxing and Labeling are first. So find a U-haul or Box City or Home Depot, or so many places in your local area that sell boxes… Boxes are cheap. Buy a box.

# Label = Enable = Be Able to Work Faster

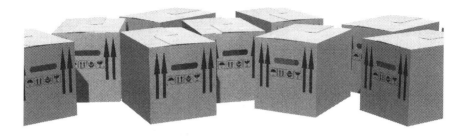

Don't throw things into your pillowcases and car, only to end up with broken, chipped or damaged items; especially when they were items you were taking with you, because it was something that you loved. When your belongings have meaning, take care of them.

**Label your boxes**. That's right: grab your child's crayons, a nice big marker, a pen, a pencil, some paint, or buy a label maker. **Just make sure you label your boxes:** dishes, kitchen, lamps, stemware, and fragile glass! Make sure your box is marked what room it goes in; and wrap things nicely in bubble wrap or tissue paper, newspaper or padding.

Make your life easy and **wrap your items and mark them properly**. Jack Canfield, in his *"Principles of Success,"* suggests an index box. He suggests you label your boxes A, B, C or 12345, etc. And every time you throw something into a box you make an index card: scuba gear box 5, snow boots box 23, so when you are looking for your snow boots, simply go to your index box and look under "S" for snow boots, and it will automatically let you know they are in box 23. This saves hours and hours of stress, and makes packing and unpacking a joy and a pleasure.

Next, **GET RID OF STUFF**. I know, I know. You love that old t-shirt, that bowling trophy, or that valentine from your crush in 2nd grade. Yet, **letting go** is part of the secret to success. One must make room for the new and wonderful things to enter their life.

George Carlin has a hysterical skit on Stress and your STUFF. Whenever you'd like to belly laugh thru your move, this is worth a viewing. You can see it anytime on YouTube. The minute you die every piece of stuff that you have ever owned belongs to someone else, so let it go… and it will help you become more Stress Free!

Another Stress-Reducer is actually having a plan. Yes, **A Plan**… do you know what room that item is going in? That's always helpful. We know so many men, thru our years of practice, who have had children. Often a man will build the baby's crib in the living room and then try to move it into the nursery. The operative word is "try" a crib does not fit thru the doorway. Every man we know, who has had this experience, has been stressed. He must then disassemble the crib and rebuild it in the room it was meant to go into – the nursery.

### *Don't give yourself extra work and stress:*

### *Know where your things are going to go!*

Next, **take care of yourself.** Moving is both mentally and physically exhausting. Rest, eat healthy food, and drink plenty of fluids. Watch your back and how you lift your items; use a dolly, ask for help, and take supplements. Remember there won't be a couch to lie on! So we need you to be up on your feet, healthy, strong and stress-free.

Another key element is to trust in your preparation: you've labeled everything, the movers are a good company and, since there are no tragedies to deal with, take pride in how well you have prepared.

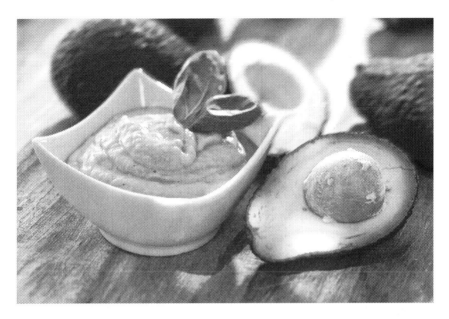

Taking care of your body is accomplished by an intake of healthy foods. Avocados are very nutritious as they contain: healthy monounsaturated fats, pantothenic acid, fiber, vitamin K, copper, folic acid, vitamin B6, potassium, vitamin E, and vitamin C.

# "Being fearless doesn't mean living a life devoid of fear, but living a life in which our fears don't hold us back."

© Lewis Publishing 2017

# CHAPTER 5

# FOUR TYPES OF STRESS

Did you know there are only **4 kinds of Stress**? That's right! Whatever kind of stress you're feeling now is one of 4 simple categories, and that stress is weighing on your life. Knowing how to deal with stress, relieving stress and relinquishing stress are easy once you know what's causing your stress; strain, pain or unhappiness. Baskin Robbins has over 31 flavors of ice cream, we have millions of diseases and illnesses, you probably have more jackets or shoes than there are avenues of stress. So today, we're going to break it down for you. Did you ever hear the expression, "*it's a cinch by the inch?*" Now we'll break it down into small, viable pieces that you can: see, feel, touch, and understand, so you too can relinquish stress from your life forever.

When stresses come up (**and they will** because that's part of living on this planet), like a rubber band, or a bow and arrow, you'll know how to manage that stress and send it on its way!

First, we have **Mental and Emotional Stress**. Do you remember the Thinking Man? We furrow our brow, rub our hands together, pace like a Bengal tiger across the floor: have sleepless nights, punch things, break things, worry, cry, rage, or retreat. We are a busy lot as a species of thinkers.

Can thinking cause and create **Mental Stress?** Yes! After all, someone discovered DNA, the cure for the measles, the airplane; and someone thought to put a man on the moon. We developed the light bulb, the computer, and when the stock market crashes; it plays with our Mental State, creating and causing what we've come to know as Stress.

First, it's our **Emotional** body and emotional life that triggers the mental stress. We all think: and feel, and care, and share, and need and want, and desire and dream, and experience all those emotions. We feel the high and lows, sorrows and losses: anticipation, drive, urges and heightened awareness to love, hate, war, crime, pain, and tragedy. Every thought is like a bell on the carnival scale, just waiting to be rung. It is here: in our thoughts, in our emotions, in our laughter, in our tears, in our worries, that mental stress comes to play. **It's important that you stay focused on the positive.**

You lost your job, so how can you feed your family? Your wife will be disappointed; the kids will go hungry! All these emotions lead to one big ball of mental exertion we have come to know as mental stress.

Will she marry me? Will he propose?

Our house was torn apart in a tornado and we lost everything. First are the tears: then the emptiness, followed by the pain fraught with helplessness, and an overwhelming sadness. How will I live? How do I go on? Then comes the wave of mental and emotional stress – they go hand in hand. Emotions fuel our mental stress. And once you learn the correlation, you can unravel the mystery of your sleepless nights and painful headaches; and together, we can relieve and relinquish your mental and emotional stress like never before.

Can you recognize that mental stress is in all of us? When we think, when we make a decision — even if it's: what to have for breakfast, or what to wear, or what to name our children, or which road to take to work. Our brains connect to our emotions and anxiety kicks in: *"I'll be late for work, there's too much traffic, I should take another road, I'll be fired or I'll never get that promotion."* The fear that jumped into the passenger seat of our car – just opened the door to mental stress.

We've all heard of **Anxiety and Tension.** Whether it's: waiting for the baby to be born, asking for a raise, speaking in public, taking an exam, getting married, racing to catch a plane, running into an old flame, losing a game, sharing holidays with your family, going to a class reunion, throwing a party, waiting in line at the supermarket – **anything and anytime where we have anxiety or tension – our bodies immediately fly into emotional stress.**

**Anger and Frustration:** From watching a boxing match, to a tire blowing on the way to work, being turned down, losing your job, someone cheating on you, injustice, not getting your way, losing money at the casino or betting of any kind, not being heard, not being seen, being abused, not having the right tools or funds to fulfill your dreams — **all of these cause anger and frustration that we feel as emotional stress.**

**Any major change in lifestyle**: making money, losing money, moving, divorce, loss of a spouse or loved one, losing a child, a sudden illness, losing agility or movement, car accidents, a house fire, flood or natural disaster, plane crashes, earthquakes or political takeovers can cause us stress.

**Our greatest gift, our mind, can and does often absolutely lead to stress.** So how do we get out of it, that constant thinking, or as we call it – stinking thinking?

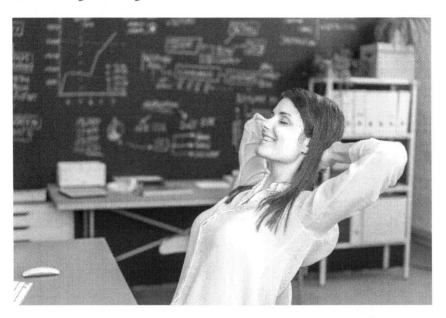

Every hour, take a 5-minute break. Take a deep breath and stretch your arms wide; then lean back, close your eyes and think of a pleasant thought for a few minutes. Then stand up and walk around your desk; bend over and try and touch your feet. Then return to your chair with fresh oxygen in your brain, ready to focus again.

**First type of stress is Emotional Stress —
relates to thinking problems**

*(see below)*

## Please Help 'I Can't Stop Thinking'

Sometimes, when you know too much, your thinking may be lead you into a bad situation with your friendships and relationships. Here's how that happened with me.

I had read an article about people who read a lot — and all of sudden it hit me — I had not been using my brain enough! So I started reading anything I could get my hands on. This led me to questioning so many things that I had been accustomed to accepting.

At work, on my lunch break, I was furiously writing down sentences that I felt were extremely important for everyone to know. However, when I would leave these little diamonds of wisdom on small pieces of paper, my efforts were not appreciated.

My co-workers resented my efforts to illuminate their minds and a bunch of them reported this to my boss. So my boss laid it on the line for me, *"Johnson, your brain is thinking way too much and it's interfering with many people in this department. It's time shape up or ship out. One more appearance of your tiny notes and you'll be fired out of a huge canon into oblivion."*

I was so depressed that I ran to the library and walked up and down the rows of books, and that wonderful smell of old pages revived me completely. Once again, I was filled with strong energy and great awareness.

So then I asked my wife what she thought of all this. Surely, she was going to back me up and support my every move. However, she just shook her head in disbelief and said: *"I know that you've been thinking, and that's why I want a divorce!"* Then her voice starting shaking and she screamed desperately, *"I'm going to my Mothers!"*

"Well, I'm going to the library," I screamed back! I needed some Albert Campus existentialism.

That's when I finally had a serious talk with myself. And I said, *"Look, I've got to come to a new decision on this matter. Will I choose my self-guided mission to educate my fellow beings? Or would I stop my brain from destroying my job, my friendships, and my marriage?"*

As I roared into the library parking lot, and got out, a poster on the building caught my attention. It read, *"Do you find that heavy thinking is ruining your life?"*

*So I sought those people out, and eventually, I joined Thinkers Anonymous. So here I am today - a* recovering thinker.

At each meeting we watch an entertaining video. Last week it was "Porky's." Afterward, we share experiences about how we avoid thinking. Listening to those testimonials has made all the difference.

**Now I'm liked at my job, and things have gotten a lot better at home. Overall, life is much better, now that I've stopped thinking.**

You will probably recognize that line. It comes from the standard Thinkers Anonymous (TA) poster. Which is why I am what I am today, a recovering thinker. I never miss a TA meeting. At each meeting we watch a non-educational video: last week it was "Porky's." Then we share experiences about how we avoid thinking since the last meeting. I still have my job, and things are a lot better at home. Life just seemed… easier, somehow, as soon as I stopped thinking.

The second category of Stress is **Thermal**. Lucky you, one doesn't happen to come across **Thermal Stress** in their daily living.

Of course the take away line in the blockbuster movie *"Frozen"* is; *"Some people are worth melting for."* Frosty the snowman has his merry song, and the wicked witch melted with a bucket of water.

Understand, you probably are not walking into meat freezers, or dog sledding in the Antarctica or visiting Santa at the North Pole today, so your chances of Thermal Stress are very slim today. However if you experience: extreme temperatures, rapid temperature changes, drowning in the ocean, being caught in a fire or explosion, (an illness that raises your temperature to an unnatural daily level), frostbite, shivering, walking on a sidewalk or hot surface, burns, being lost while camping, hiking or rappelling (*rope climbing; a descent from a cliff or wall in which one slides down an anchored rope and applies friction in order to control one's speed*), being caught in storms or tornados, high winds, or spilling your coffee on your lap, **all create Thermal Stress**.

Today there are amazing new techniques to keep a body frozen in a high-tech-induced coma state in order to recover the mind and the body's functionality after drowning or a trauma. This amazing technique is safely able to return the body to its healthy, natural state. Life-saving tools for fire victims are now available and medicine has much to offer to bring our fevers down and return us to optimal health, freedom and a stress-free life.

The 3rd avenue of Stress is **Physical**. That's correct. We are not talking about some new fangled sexual position. We are talking about: growing pains, breaking your arm, falling out of a tree, getting whacked in the face with a hockey stick, arthritis, heart disease, gum disease, poor posture, scoliosis, being overweight, or anorexic, or bulimic. In addition, if you experience: not sleeping properly, poor eyesight, loss of hearing or senses, surgeries, hip replacements, having a baby, back pain, knee pain, rotator cuff pain, incontinence, Crohns disease, a stroke, loss of a limb, running a marathon or triathlon, football, white water rafting, hitting your thumb with the hammer, burning your hand on the pot, slipping on the ice, **and sexual incompetence can all lead to Physical Stress.** Physical stress has many ways to either cause or alleviate the pain, problem or barrier. We'll explore each and every effective method as you turn thru the pages of this book.

The 4th avenue to Stress is more common in our daily life than we realize, and that is **Chemical Stress**. That's right, have you ever read your cereal label? Have you stood by the gas pump thinking the smell was making you sick or that you felt nauseous, weak or faint? Have you driven behind a bus or **car emitting fumes**? (Studies have linked exhaust from diesel engines to cancers.)

Have you found yourself in a roaring nightclub, or a sports bar with a **smoke-filled** room? Or maybe your parents or grandparents smoked, or you had a college stint filled with bongs and substances that wreaked havoc with your brain.

Have **Stimulants** like **coffee or tea** ruled your life? Is your diet filled with food additives and sugar-based products? Do you have a 'healthy food' pattern or are you having chocolate pancakes for breakfast? Any unbalanced diet can send us into a chemical spin. Diabetic and **chocolate addicts** can all tell you about mood swings, emotional agony and — boy, do they know about stress!

Food is perhaps, one of the hardest disciplines to maintain because the most difficult part is dealing with our emotions. **Comfort eating can be displaced by higher goals that you desire.**

A good recommendation is that you find a positive reason for following a good eating pattern that is free from emotions. For example, one good affirmation can be, *"If I eat better, then I can focus better at work, and that will bring me a good chance of a promotion!"*

**Alcohol** puts us in a wild intangible zone. Ask an alcoholic, where did they leave their car? Was it in the middle of the road? Were cops chasing them as they weaved down the street? How did it feel waking up on the floor somewhere, or in a stranger's bed, and being completely unaware of how they got there? Or how about when they were falling down and somehow, injured themselves, or hurt others? All of these scenarios are absolutely heap loads of stress.

Have you ever gone hiking, or climbed a mountain, and the altitude had you feeling like you were floating or dizzy; or maybe you had a headache? **High altitudes** very often put the body into immediate chemical stress.

**Drugs** and even our **prescribed medications** can stress-out our bodies and stress-out our internal organs. An upset tummy at a kid's birthday party after pizza and ice cream is an indication of a stressed-out stomach. Our other organs, bowels and digestive track can be overtaxed when we consume high quantities of medication or recreational drugs and substances.

The good news is all of these avenues can be avoided. Imagine a grand map to happiness and satisfaction and take another road. **Yes, you can be Stress Free!**

# CHAPTER 6

# FROM THE GROUND UP STRESS CAN MELT AWAY

Oh, my feet… my poor, poor feet; bet your life a waitress really earns her pay. I've been on my feet, my poor, poor feet, hour after hour today.

The musical *"Working,"* features this song where the waitress stops and rubs her feet while she sings the song. I bet when your feet hurt, you don't feel much like singing. From teachers, to sales clerks, to military personal, to shop keepers: from security to coaches, from bank tellers to crossing guards, so many jobs in today's world keep us on our feet and often wracked with pain.

How come so many romantic movies entice us with the rubbing of a partner's foot as the way to fall in love?

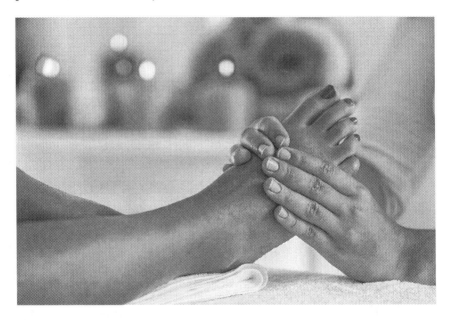

Do you know how many bones are in your feet? I bet it's like counting jelly beans in a jar for a contest and a prize. There are actually 28 bones, 33 joints and 107 ligaments that make up the structure of your foot, and only 1 needs to hurt – and it can drive you wild! Have you ever stubbed your toe, and then jumped around your living room for ten minutes? Have you tripped over a toy, worn new shoes on a convention hall floor, or gone dancing for hours in shoes only Cinderella could wear? If our feet could talk, they are our abused children. Child services would quickly whisk our feet away for neglect and abuse, if they saw how we treated our most precious element.

Even the neighborhood piano teacher is peddling away with their foot. At what point do our feet get a break; and how can we relieve the stress?

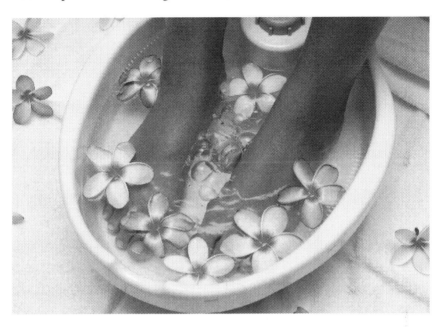

Born free… somehow we have the impression that running barefoot on the grass will take us back to our youth and help us grown big and strong. Actually it puts grass stains on the carpet and tracks mud into your house! Running around in bare feet is not the answer. Did you know that just walking barefoot (on a hard, flat surface) exposes the foot to extra intensity on the ground? Now who needs extra intensity? Not you or I, (maybe a horror film writer), yet certainly not the foot.

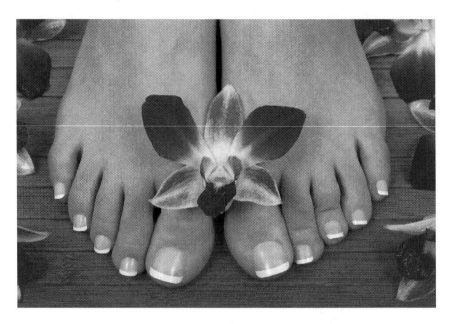

Our ancestors were barefoot. They ran around with spears and climbed mountains without any shoes. They walked on ancient soil and they tilled the earth. Yes, but there were no sidewalks, concrete convention center floors, tile hospital corridors; or badly made stairs to run upon. They didn't have chemicals and pesticides in the grass and they definitely didn't have Jimmy Choo Shoes. Natural earth had a 'give' to it that went with the body, and it acted as a springboard for life and energy, from the planet in which we lived. Walking on hard and manufactured surfaces, over time, corrupts the foot and causes major problems in our life. The fatty tissue is literally pushed aside and creates a low-level inflammation on the underside of the metatarsal bones. (Now doesn't that sound mighty painful? You remember the first time you counted a baby's toes: 1-2-3-4-5-6-7-8-9-10 little chubby toes that went to the market and guess what? They wore shoes!

**Statistic: The average American walks 18,000 steps a day**

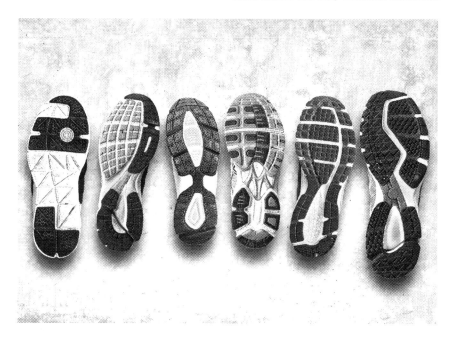

## Well Padded Shoes Help Sore Feet

When you're in your 20's and 30's, you may not notice a huge difference. Only trust us; your mind is overriding the problem. In just a few short years, your feet will no longer be your friends. They are angry and sad and frustrated that you let them run over the hot, cement sidewalk from the beach to your car. Or that you ran over the pebbles and rocks, when you were camping, or that you walked over the chemically-treated grass to grab your mail and your newspaper. And then trapped them in inappropriate shoes to dance, ski, skate, or impress your co-workers. When your feet get mad, you will feel their anger; and you will know that the abuse and its effects have just begun.

But I wear **shoes** you say. I throw on flip-flops so my feet aren't bare. **Flip flops are naked feet without any protection or support.** It's like going braless in a t-shirt. You get the idea. Often when wearing flip–flops, our toes are gripping with fear. That motion creates what we've come to know as **Hammer Toes**. Not a pretty picture in society today. Also flip–flops that require you to grip them with your toes, overtime, will cause an irritation to your tendons. It's called **tendonitis**.

Imagine this is something that we can avoid entirely in our life. Now that's a relief.

**Men's shoes** were not designed for health and happiness. Imagine a tie wrapped tightly around your neck. How comfortable is that? Probably the same maniacal fellow had a hand in the creation of designing what we've come to know as the man's shoe. What about **Men's loafers?** They may look comfortable yet; they have very little padding for the feet.

An easy solution is simply adding a **cushioned insert** and life immediately gets better. Drug Stores, sporting goods stores, and even some clothing and department stores; carry a wide variety of pads for your pleasure, comfort and delight. Remember to select an insert specifically designed for dress shoes, when you first buy your shoes!

Which ones should I buy? Since I'm not at the department store with you, I'll use my magic crystal ball and I'd say, choose the one that is made of **synthetic rubber (neoprene**, etc.); which will hold up over time. Today you can even go online and purchase an insert that will save you years of stress and headaches. Now that's the greatest investment of all.

**Women's shoes:** Ah... the secret of sexy, allure, enticement, and beauty. What little girl hasn't tried on a pair of her mother's **high heel shoes** and trotted around the house. What fantasy lies in the minds of women and men, around women's shoes? They are the focal point of our ads; timeless beauty, our fairytales and even Mother Hubbard lived in a shoe. Women build closets for their shoes, they will save months of paychecks for the designer shoe of the day. Statistics show a man will pick up an item that a woman had dropped quicker and respond more often if a woman is wearing high heels compared to flat shoes. High-heeled bedroom slippers are ensemble with negligees and Victoria Secret has its runway models in high heels and underwear. How come we sell bras and panties with high-heeled shoes? A better question is how come women are attracted to buy these outfits.

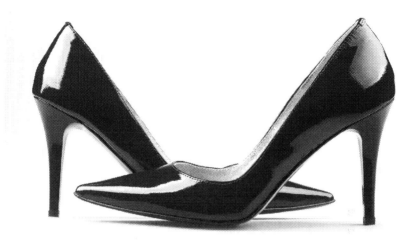

Women's shoes were designed after the ancient Chinese slippers; where women's feet were painfully bound and held captive for men's pleasure and delight. That binding forced to accentuate the calf, which is what we find alluring and provocative with women in high heel shoes today. Yes, high heel shoes accentuate the calf, **however they do it while destroying the foot.** A mere thin 4 to 5-inch heel can cause knee, calf and ankle problems for years to come. High heel shoes, just like in men's shoes, offer little or no padding, which we all know is a danger in itself.

Next, the height is a playground for **ankle twisting.** And **tendons** and **ligaments** are often so compromised they may fear for their little lives, as they're carefully just barely hanging on. The foot wobbles and it is forced to move back and forth in the shoe. Have you ever walked behind a woman in high heel shoes? It looks like her foot is going to come falling out, and flying out of the shoe, leaving her tumbling to the ground in front of you. Yet, somehow, she balances and walks unevenly as we worry for her safety; not to mention her foot catching up second by second to the shoe and it's movement.

Have you ever made of list of shoe designers? That's right, they are mostly men. Designing Shoes and Designer Stilts for a women's foot, think about that for a minute. Not to mention, the elevation alone can cause major **back problems** by putting undue pressure on the sacrum. Did you know the elevation takes up to 7 times the pressure on your toes and their **metatarsal padding?** (It is located directly on the sole of your foot, just below your toes.) Did you feel it? Yes, there!

I'd suggest just as I have for the men… If you're going to don those sexy shoes, then cushion them with an adequate pad or padding to protect your feet. **Flat shoes** for woman can also use some padding to protect those tender tendons and your shimmering, precious and beautifully manicured toes.

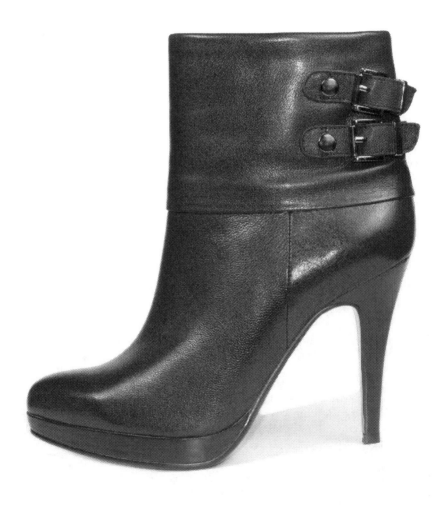

**Ballerina Girl!** Who hasn't been swept away by the Snow Queen, or Clair, in the "Nutcracker"? Women on point are elegant, graceful and the "dream come true." They live in the fantasy world and the Prince throws them high in the air and twirls them around o**n their toes**. Ouch, yes!

They stand directly on a metal box on their toes. If you've never been a ballerina and men go with me here, they actually stand on a metal box. They sell padding such as lamb's wool and little bunny fur pads for teenage girls but, **mature professional dancers** forsake the padding to feel the balance and they stand directly in narrow slipper on a metal box. **Bunions, Hammer toes** and a variety of foot problems develop for dancers of all stages and figure skaters alike. **Cramped toes** in "any" shoe leads to pressure on the joint of the big toe, and a crushing effect on the smaller ones. Very often painful deformities develop such as bunions. This is known as a **dancer's foot**. Like a warrior, the battle scars of the victory leave a lifelong and lasting impression that can be avoided with care, awareness, and a little padding and room.

**Pedicures** – Get your feet pampered. Men and Women; let someone care for your feet. When you have: hard, rough, ugly **calluses** that they are muscling off with every visit, or when you have big, **dry, rough, or cracked heels,** and your foot looks like the picture of stress, you might want to add some **Vitamin A**. One of our mentors, Dr. Jonathan Wright, told us that heavy, heel calluses were a sign of long-term vitamin A deficiency. He recommended vitamin A (not beta-carotene), supplementation for individuals with this problem. He said that you should start with 75,000 units of vitamin A per day until the calluses are gone. Then you can decrease your dose to a "maintenance amount" of 10,000 to 15,000 units per day. That high level of oxygen will make your calluses, and tough skin, go away.

For **Sore tired feet,** give them a treat. Take them to your home bakery. No not pie, cake or strudel. Just grab the **old fashion rolling pin** and roll back and forth over the feet. Now that's a delightful treat and a surefire way to make your feet happy today!

**Cold Feet** – Have you ever gotten into bed with someone who has cold feet, and you jump so high, you almost bump your head on the ceiling? Well maybe that didn't happen, but it made you jump and in the moment you said something comforting to your spouse or loved one like; *"Geez, do you have cold feet!"* Your cold feet are a sign of **poor circulation and STRESS**.

**Water** is known as the essence of life. **Warm footbaths** increase circulation and relieve the built up of tension of the foot. A warm footbath with **Epsom salts,** brimming with **magnesium,** can easily penetrate the skin to relax the muscles, tendons and ligaments, while adding a luxurious and pleasurable experience to your day. Even better than water are the new, **infrared foot warmers**. Top Notch research has shown amazing results and these delightful warmed and cozy footie's can penetrate your foot even deeper than water, relaxing those muscles and having you well on your way to stress-free living.

Today we have lovely paved roads, streets, sidewalks and highways. As a matter of fact, we actually complain when a sidewalk is cracked or a road has some wear and tear upon it. Long ago, back in our fairytale life, we had cobblers and we had cobblestone streets. Did you know that cobblestones *can actually reverse aging?* What? That's right! The cobblestones actually elicit a very therapeutic response. Just by comparing cobblestones to walking rectangular, you'll be amazed at the effect, and health of the feet, and their life patterns.

Indians wore moccasins to not only protect the foot; it was also to feel the earth and those 3-5 inch river stones, which helped our ancestors and forefather's muscles on their feet and arches to stay proper, healthy and aligned.

The creation and invention of cobblestones follows Chinese holistic medicine and the use and principles of Reflexology. The cobblestones work like acupuncture and acupressure to stimulate, and to regulate, those imperative acupuncture points on the bottom of the foot. Research has shown not only vast improvement in circulation and in foot function; walking on cobblestones has proved highly effective in reducing blood pressure and promoting healthier living. And this fact means that even walking on bumpy Mother Earth performs a similar, beneficial function.

In a pilot program at the Oregon Research Institute (in Eugene, Oregon), Dr. Li, Ph.D., and his colleagues showed significant measured improvements **in just 30 - 60 minutes, 3 times a week from adults ranging from 60 - 92** in both mental and physical health by just walking on the cobblestones.

Today we can purchase **cobblestone mats,** which are very healing and especially effective for aging and elderly feet. A world of paradise awaits you in a simple purchase of a cobblestone product that can do wonders for the modern foot of today. Of course, you could always take a vacation to a historic town and have a walk about, and not only improve your feet but it can also improve your mental, spirit and soul state, not to mention the quality of your life.

### The art of being happy lies in the power of extracting happiness from common things.

Okay we've talked about sore feet, what about **crooked feet**? You know that classic Greek foot, where the second toe is longer than the big toe because the balance has shifted. Or even the pigeon toe or the duck foot, and we often see ballerina's who walk in turnout. Would you drive a car with crooked tires? Imagine if the tires on your car were heading in opposite directions, or if one tire was larger than the other, what would happen? Would it throw the balance off? Absolutely! How would you drive? You would need a re-alignment, well so does your foot. The same way your tires need air; **your body needs silica**. You may be lacking in something as simple as **Vitamin D**.

**Bunions**… onions… peel back the layers of foot problems and bunions are lurking just waiting to ruin your day! Walk down the aisle of any supermarket, drug store, and right before your eyes are products, there are shelves of products for **corns, calluses and bunions**. We get frustrated trying on shoes, or donning sandals or strappy shoes because of our bunions. Those mountainous problems that ride alongside our feet, making it impossible to properly fit into shoes — not to mention they're ugly and often people will hide their feet in heavy socks or boots pretending they're not there — just lurking waiting for us to cry out in pain. Many people have been offered **surgery;** yet they choose to stow their feet away like war prisoners, giving them little light and freedom and torturing them along the way. Now what kind of life is that for your precious little feet?

Your big toe is struggling and turning laterally just to maintain your balance. You're binding it and hiding it, instead of facing the problem head on and alleviating not only the bunion issue, but also **balance, posture** and a healthy stress-free living.

Maybe you just need an **orthotic**. If you looked at your heel you would have a triangle across your foot coming to the Achilles tendon. Is it straight? That angle determines the type of orthotic needed. Just a soft insert can literally change: your happiness, health, freedom, sensuality, passion, pleasure, joy and quality of life.

Even getting the **rubberband from the broccoli** and attaching it to your big toes, and stretching your toes wide open, can feel wonderful and make a world of difference to happier and healthier feet.

**Exercise your feet**. That's right. Get on a trampoline or buy a home mini tramp. Bouncing is a great way to exercise your feet and it also improves your heart, muscles, ligaments and your energy.

You know when you hear music and you naturally have the urge to move, your body loves moving. Help it; let it bounce often. **Bounce** when you're brushing your teeth or washing your face. Bounce while the shower water gets hot or the washing machine is filling up for its cycle. Just by rising up and down on your toes or doing a few squats works wonders. Trust us! Your body will love you for this! How about during those commercial breaks? Instead of running to the kitchen for more chips, you can use that time to jump in a few **exercises for your feet**. There are 6-7 commercial breaks in an hour. Making this a healthy habit allows exercise to easily become part of your daily life with little effort and tremendous results that will have you grateful, exuberant and exhilarated for years.

**Runners and Athletes** this is for you. When you run regularly or participate in sports, you are already prone to straining the ligaments of the foot. This is the tissue that connects bone to bone, which extends from your heel, through the arch of your foot – all the way to the padding.

One day you may wake up and experience **pain in the heel of the foot** as you start to walk (*Plantar fascilitis*). The morning is usually the most painful time — the Plantar ligament has tightened over the night while you were sleeping — tricky ligament, why couldn't it take a break like the rest of your body?

**The Art of the Towel**: We've always been amazed at the multiplicity of uses for a simple, hand towel. From sweat to sanitary bedding, from a pillow to a life-saving tourniquet, a **towel** is an invaluable item in an athlete's arsenal and toolbox. One of the greatest stretches of all time is executed with a common hand towel. Of course, if it has the name of your favorite health club, sports team, hotel or vacationed city, somehow it seems to have more power and versatility than ever before.

Here's how it works: you sit on the floor with your legs extended in front of you, and you should feel better already. Now gently wrap the towel in a loop around the top half of the foot, almost as if you were lassoing your toes. Now securely grasp both ends of the towel in each hand. Using only your arm strength, you can slightly pull your foot towards you… ah!

Doesn't that feel better? You should feel a wonderful stretch in the instep of your foot. Yes, that's where the **plantar ligament** is located and you have just relieved the temporary stress of your foot in one small and simple move.

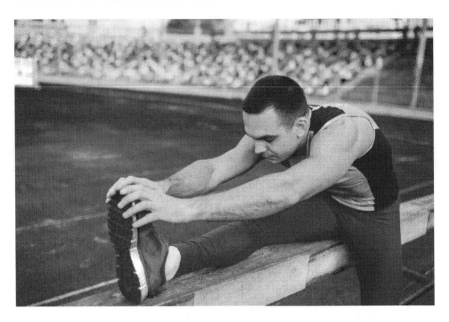

**Although the pictured stretch above is a little different than the towel stretch, it is the same principle.** If this gentle stretch does relieve your pain, than try this next one.

The **"ice bottle" remedy** is also recommended by physical therapists: fill up an 8-inch plastic bottle and leave about 2" empty. (Do not use a glass bottle!) Then place the plastic bottle in the freezer. Each morning, take the bottle out of the freezer and place the ice bottle on a rug. Sit in a simple straight back chair near the bottle. Gently lower your painful, bare foot onto the bottle. (If the cold is too intense, place a light, cotton shirt over the bottle to reduce the cold.) The most important area is the instep of your foot, right where you feel the pain. Roll the bottle back and forth slowly with your foot, allowing the cold to chill the instep and heel of your foot.

Often late in the day or in the evening, your foot will feel the pressure of the day and the irritation will veer itself as pain at the most inopportune time: just when you are winding down, heading out on a hot date, or off to a dinner meeting to close that million dollar deal. What if tonight was the father daughter dance or your daughter's wedding?

What if you finally made time for that romantic getaway to Paris, and the night stroll caught you by surprise as your foot was engulfed in pain. **You can prevent this condition from happening when you wear shoes with sturdy arch supports and have adequate padding under your feet.**

Fun Foot Facts:

**For a 150 lb. person, each foot bears 127,000 pounds of pressure while walking a mile.**

**In an average lifetime the feet log more than 100,000 miles. Now that's a lot of walking!**

**Every athlete knows about Achilles — In Greek Mythology he was a hero.** What lead to his downfall and ultimately to his death was the arrow that was shot to his heel, which shows the vulnerabilities in us all.

**Proper Stretching** can easily prevent tightness in the calves as well as alleviate tightness and vulnerability to the **Achilles tendon** (a tough band of fibrous tissue that connects the calf muscles to the heel bone).

A great stretch can be achieved in just minutes. A proper *Runners Stretch* begins at an arms distance from the wall. While facing the wall, you can lean against the wall with both hands making contact, now step back with one foot, and make sure to align the back foot with the front foot. You should feel supported, aligned and completely safe and relaxed. Now slowly… lean forward, slight bend and flex your elbows. This feels good already doesn't it? Now shift your weight from the back foot to the front foot. As the heel of the back foot remains in contact with the floor, you are stretching the calf muscle and Achilles tendon. Hold the stretch for 20 seconds. **Stay steady – No Bouncing!** And don't forget to breathe.

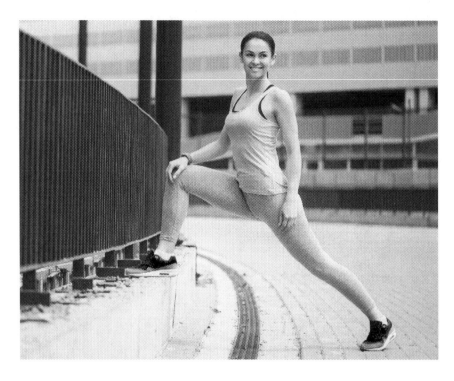

This picture is a little different than the one described. **Her hands should be on the railing** and her back foot should be straight.

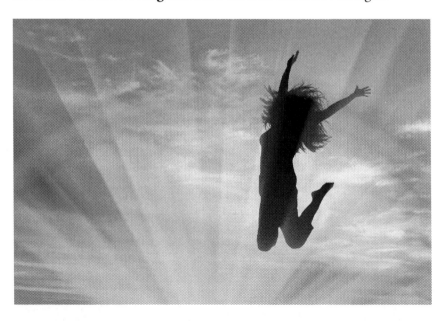

# CHAPTER 7

# WALK OFF THE PAIN

## Walk like a Man — Talk like a Man — Walk like a Man my son...

When you walk thru the storm, hold your head up high and don't be afraid of the dark. How many songs and stories teach us about the strength and the power of walking?

Babies get up and they start to walk, they toddle and they fall down. We do not learn to walk; we learn to balance. Walking comes naturally. **Walking is considered the most fundamental human motor activity and what do we do?** We sit at a desk: or we watch TV, or we lie in bed, or we drive our cars, or we lounge by our pools, but our heart really wants us to walk. We used to walk to the television to change the channel. Now we even have remote controls or a master switch.

> **"My grandmother started walking five miles a day when she was sixty. She's ninety-seven now, and we don't know where the heck she is."**
>
> **— Ellen DeGeneres**

We used to walk to school. How many grandparents and elders tell the story of how they use to walk to school in the snow? It's a fabled part of our lives; yet today, the average person is sedentary, complacent and just plain lazy. How many people complain about walking, from the parking lot to the mall, the restaurant or even to the gym?

Did you know walking is miraculous? Walking can provide **stress reduction** on the heart, the organs and even **increase muscle strength**. Just the swinging motion alone of your arms and legs (**cross-crawling**), rebalances your **brain's electrical activity**, which helps your brain to perform in an optimum fashion.

Yes! You can **lose weight** by walking... this doesn't mean that you should rush out and order a pizza, but the fast-paced motion is a natural way to reduce stress and burn fat. Brisk walking can actually turn off excess "Cortisol Release" **and prevents extra belly fat on your stomach, love handles and your waistline.**

What a great secret to a healthy body and a healthy life!

Boys used to walk girls to their classrooms; we strolled through parks and towns and we walked over to our neighbor's house just to say hello. In as little as 8 minutes-a-day, you can be benefiting your body and showing measurable results, simply by putting one foot in front of the other.

Imagine an airport and all the people are on the people movers instead of simply walking to their gate. Elevators and escalators replace our sturdy, durable and dependable stairs and even our mail gets delivered thru our computer so we don't have to walk to the curb eagerly anticipating a letter, or good news in our postal box.

Before all this high tech technology, we didn't need Brazilian Butt videos to give us a high, lifted and taut backside. We had sidewalks and stairs that lifted our derrieres, and our cheeks on our face were also rosy and bright from the fresh air and exercise. We always looked, healthy, fit and alive.

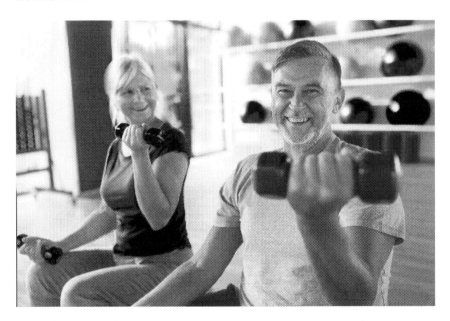

Research after research has been done, and each and every time, guess what? The walkers were healthier, happier and more vibrant, radiant and more fit than the group that was not walking on a regular basis.

From Japan to John Hopkins, researchers, doctors and scientists alike will confirm **20 – 30 minutes of walking a day can vastly improve your health.**

Babies start to walk yet; first they crawl. That motion from the opposite hand to the opposite knee feeds our **neurological pathways** (through what is called our *cross-crawling motion*). Often when someone has been severely injured or even often in stroke cases or accidents alike, a physical therapist will teach a *cross-crawling* motion to regenerate that part of the brain, and the motion and impulse to move forward. When we walk, our arms swing naturally back-and-forth. And as we move our legs across the floor, we develop the opposite sides of the brain simultaneously. And that pumping motion keeps our bodies and our brains in flow, and optimum motion. Hard shoes often hinder the **pumping action** and restrict us from our growth and thriving action. Mind your body — it is there to support you. If you can assist it in its desires you can lead a happy, healthy and stress free life.

> *A specialist in the obesity field James Levine, M.D., PhD, commented: "You don't have to join a gym, you don't have to check your pulse. You just have to switch off the TV, get off the sofa and go for a walk."*

Even as we shared the problems of walking on a chemically induced lawn, or a sidewalk brimming with dangers, and volatile landmines, in order **to ground yourself,** we encourage you to **walk on the earth**. Earth not dirt... you know "earth" where flowers grow and plants grow supplying minerals and vitamins, and nature and sunshine bask in life and the essence of healing of all that is. That earth can be very grounding for your body and your soul. **Walking on the sand at the beach** can also be equally healing and therapeutic.

Did you know that electrons from the earth have anti-aging properties? **Every known symptom of every known disease comes from a Free Radical. A Free Radical is a chemical minus an electron.** Therefore, every known symptom of every known disease is the loss of an electron. So imagine how easy it is to absorb those electrons and to drastically improve your state of health, and your overall wellness, by simply taking a walk!

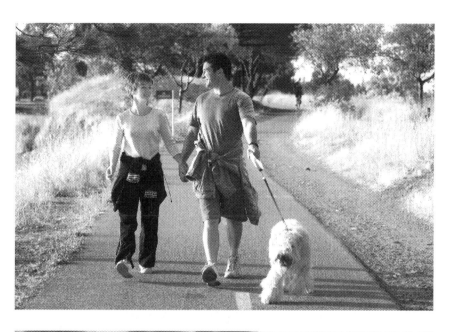

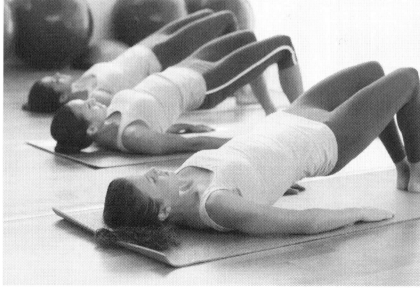

There is an old parable that illustrates an important philosophical and religious truth that applies to all of us. Once a man had a dream that illuminated his mind. In this dream, he's walking on a sandy beach with God, and notices two footprints as they are walking. He interprets this to mean that God in walking with him as his protector.

At the same time, the man sees his life revealed before him. Soon, he is startled to see only one set of footprints that corresponds to the worst period of his life. He immediately turns and bursts out, and accuses God of abandoning him in his time of need.

Then God, in his most benevolent way, answers him saying that he always loves him and he would never desert him. Finally says, **it was my footprints as I carried you through your darkest times.**

Even in this parable, we are told that God walks. That's a powerful thought and certainly there's something to be said for walking.

Walking even in small increments can be stress reducing. Imagine winding down from a hard day at work, or even having 5 minutes of solitude and time to think away from your kids. Nothing cures anger faster than walking away; taking a walk to clear your head or just getting some fresh air – and with a new perspective on how deeply God loves you.

This reaffirms our need to realize that we are always connected to the Divinity and that love is the most aspect of life.

> *"If you seek creative ideas go walking. Angels whisper to a man when he goes for a walk."*
>
> **— Raymond I. Myers**

Walking in any amount can **reduce stress, pain, tightness, tension and fatigue.** Imagine walking on stage to win an award, graduating from a university, traveling with a parade; or even strolling to see the Christmas lights in the windows of holiday delight. Walking is enchanting, powerful, energizing and just phenomenal for almost every scenario in your life.

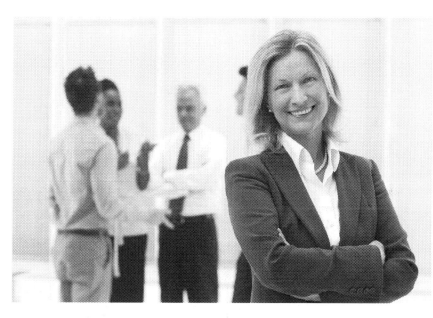

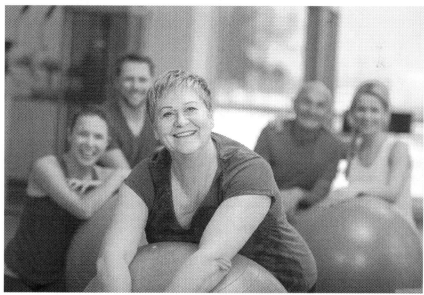

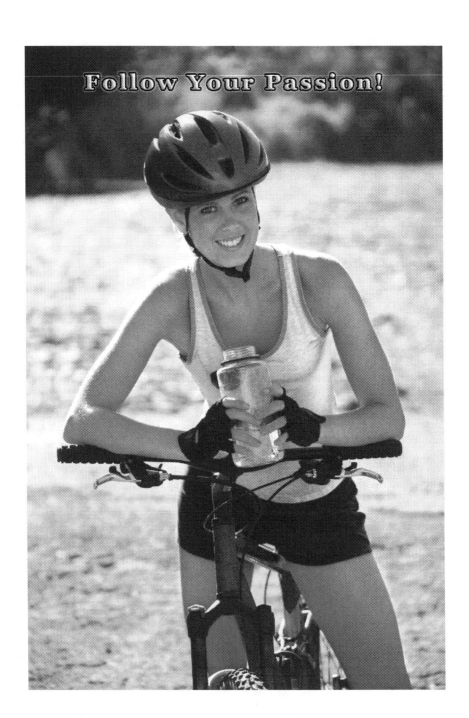
Follow Your Passion!

# CHAPTER 8

# HELPFUL HINTS

## <u>Helpful Hints</u>

**Bones** need Sulfa (sulfanilamide acid) and Nutrients to survive and thrive. Our bodies long for: **Silica, Vitamin C, Lysine, L-proline, Vitamin D, Magnesium, Calcium, Phosphate, Vitamin K and Sulfa.** Although many nutrients can be found in our food, depending upon your diet and your lifestyle, one or more of these **vitamins and nutrients** may be lacking from your overall wellness and life. Companies and products like our **Prime Longevity** (http://primelongevity.com), and Alkagenics (http://www.alpha-genics.com) have many options for supplementing your health, and adding primary and necessary functionality to our bodies, systems and our thriving happy lives.

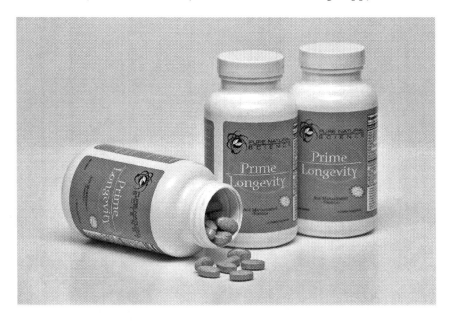

**Prime Longevity is the most powerful anti-aging formula on the market**

Further information, dosage and usage can easily be found on our **website http://primelongevity.com**

# CHAPTER 9

# THE SOUND OF SILENCE

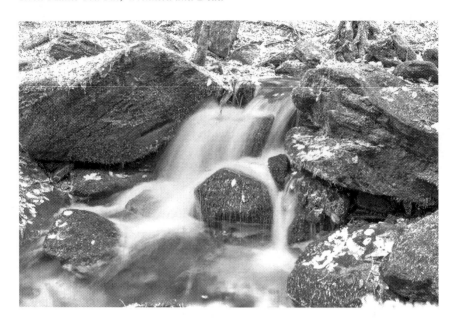

Who is aging, asked the wise owl? "Not I," said Pooh. Life in forest is carefree and magic. The birds flutter their wings, the trees rustle, the wind whispers; and the rain whooshes from the sky. Brooks share their secrets; waterfalls cascade with a symphony of rhythm, and each step in the forest is like an unlocked treasure, as your foot kisses the earth.

Songbirds sing to their hearts delight; and coyotes howl at the bright moon. Every living creature shows a sign of life from their scurrying sounds, to the fish coming to the surface to say hello. Each melodic voice is giving us a hint and the gift of life.

We used to cringe when a wrong note was played on the piano, or a child learned to the play the trumpet or the drums. When a trash can fell over, or the mop hit the floor, creaky stairs were a bother, and the rumble of a steam engine would set our heart soaring. Music would flow into the city streets from the clubs, and natives would dance around raging fires, with ancient chants in glow of the night.

Choirs would lift our spirits and the sound of children laughing could fill our hearts with glee and unspoken happiness forever more.

A car engine was seduction for a teenage boy and the words *"I love you"* were all we wanted to hear.

Today's world offers sounds like never before: loud booms, gun shots, blaring speakers, planes and jets, and washing machines and dryers with bells to let you know the cycle is complete.

Blenders and microwaves: trash trucks and sirens, cell phones in our ears and ear plugs to listen to our favorite tunes, Hi-definition TV's, and motorcycles that could stop your heart with their fierce maniacal roar.

Jack hammers and drills, even our cars make loud beeping sounds every time we back out of our driveways. Blow dryers and alarm systems, leaf blowers and car horns that honk just because someone is impatient or rushing thru their day. School bells, morning alarms and alarms on our phone just to remind us to take a call: war games, video games, gargantuan computers and copiers.

Remember when bubble gum made a snap or popcorn would pop, or when we would cheer for a home run or a winning goal? Now stadiums are so loud you can barely talk to the person next to you.

Did you know that it is estimated that 20 million Americans have suffered permanent – that is, correct – **permanent damage** to **their hearing** from **loud noise**? That's amazing.

Researchers believe that the state of our hearing worldwide is fading away at a considerable rapid speed but why, and what can we do about it?

We laugh at the Verizon commercials, *"Can you hear me now?"*

However can you hear me today? Can you hear me when I am right next to you in a car, across the table in a restaurant, when you are sitting next to me at a show: or even in our kitchen when I am making you a morning smoothie or grinding your coffee beans to start your day?

Statistics are staggering… Noise volumes of **80 decibels (and below) are classified safe** for all adults. A decibel is simply a unit for measuring the intensity of sound. So how intense is the sound in your life?

Frightening yet true, anything over this limit can cause **severe and permanent damage**. Even at 91 decibels for more than 2 hours, 100 decibels more than 15 minutes… yes 15 minutes or 120 decibels at 9 seconds is wrecking havoc with your hearing and with your life.

Have you ever jumped at a loud sound like a speaker screeching or music blaring at an unbearable volume? Have you lost your teenager to headphones, video games, or the music of today — where not only the volume explodes — but also the words and lyrics can be painful to hear as well? Simple subways: trains, diesel engines, and chain saws can measure 100 decibels. 30 minutes alone can cause a significant hearing loss.

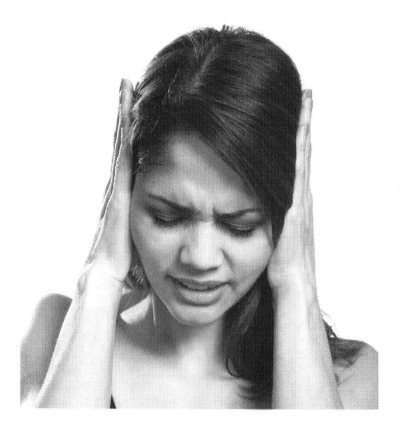

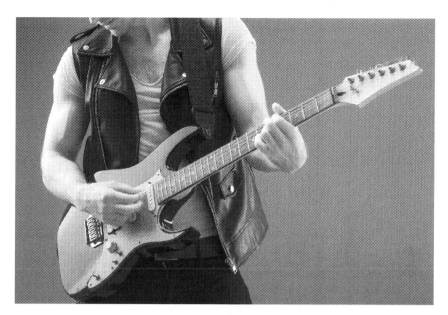

**Rock Concerts and blaring music speakers at 120 decibels** or even **IPOD ear buds**, which pump music or sound directly into your ear buds can cause quicker permanent damage than almost anything else in today's modern world. Six minutes — **yes, 6 minutes of sports arena noise equals 81 times the daily noise limit.** What!!! So what can you do?

When listening to music did you realize that you have choice? **Noise canceling ear buds,** or **Noise canceling earphones** are always an option. By blocking out extraneous background noise, listeners can even enjoy intense rock music at a lower overall volume. That's wonderful news for today's ears.

Researchers will tell us that with the frequency of modern high volume exposure, our young people now have hearing impairments 2½ times that of their grandparents. Wouldn't we rather have 2½ % more wisdom, or financial growth or health or opportunity of happiness and success?

## Tinnitus is the Result of Damaged Hearing

Many of us think that hearing loss is only a modern affliction. However, many greats of their day also experienced this terrible condition:

The great artist **Michelangelo** suffered with **Tinnitis** affliction as his writing shows, *"A spider's web is hidden in one ear, and in the other, a cricket sings throughout the night."* And while Tinnitus can be hard to explain to others, it certainly can drive people to despair.

> *"Hearing Loss is a terrible thong because it cannot be repaired."*
> *Pete Townsend*

A large majority of us are familiar with the rock band "The Who" and Pete Townsend is the brains behind it, as he has penned all of their hit songs. Nowadays, he is a vocal advocate of protecting one's hearing. At 120 decibels, rock bands blow you away with their energy as well as blowing out your hearing.

Here are some famous people who have this terrible affliction: Beethoven, Charles Darwin, Vincent Van Gogh, Howard Hughes, Rush Limbaugh, Steve Martin, David Letterman, Eric Clapton, Phil Collins, Ronald Regan, Barbra Streisand, Neil Young, Huey Lewis, Jeff Beck and Gerard Butler.

Between 40 million to 50 million Americans have *some degree of tinnitus*, often accompanied by some hearing loss. This condition is commonly brought on by **damage to the ears through exposure to loud noise**.

Tinnitus produces a constant high–pitched: whining, buzzing, or hissing sound, or maybe a rattling in the ears that is not only annoying; it is a persistent stress creator in daily life.

Nowadays, It's so common to see young people in their teens or twenties walking around with "earbuds" in their ears, constantly listening to loud music. And for the home, many also use state-of-the-art earphones that cost around $250-$300. All of this is seriously damaging to young people's hearing. After the music is over, many will experience a ringing or buzzing in their ears for a short period of time. Have you ever experienced this? This is a sign of the early stages of tinnitus – a precursor of what is called **noise-induced hearing loss.**

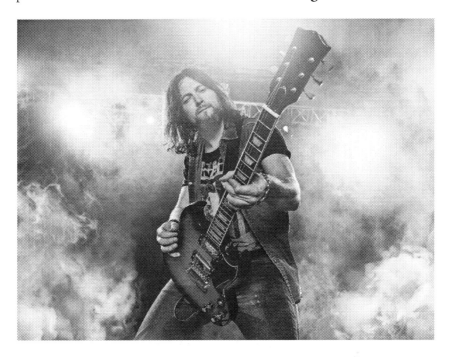

Imagine a sound that seems to be coming from the outside yet it's being created inside your world within your own sensory system. Isn't that something you'd like to avoid?

Even wearing an easy **Sponge Earplug** can reduce the noise level by 32 percent. Everything can be clear and perfect while you're still protecting your ears with any damaging or long-term effects.

Today's technology has its accolades and winners and along that line we now have **Neoprene Earplugs**. These denser earplugs can be used to protect your ears at sporting events, rock concerts, the loud clang of heavily barbells at the gym, even at loud action films or anywhere where the sound levels explode and can cause irrevocable repair.

Here you can prevent that forever annoying ringing in your ears, and you can still hear the music with impeccable sound while being able to converse freely with the person next to you. Now that's Stress-Free!

Foam is long since been associated with rest, relaxation and pleasure; foam mattresses alone have swept the nation in comfort and delight. A **foam earplug** that can block at least 32 percent can be used readily when working with power tools or loud machines. What a life saver when adding a room to your house, building a babies nursery, redoing your kitchen, adding a sun room or sun deck, or even building that tree house to retreat and stow away. Even machines registering at 85 decibels can be lowered to 53 using foam earplugs, which is completely an acceptable level and will add to your journey of Living Stress-Free.

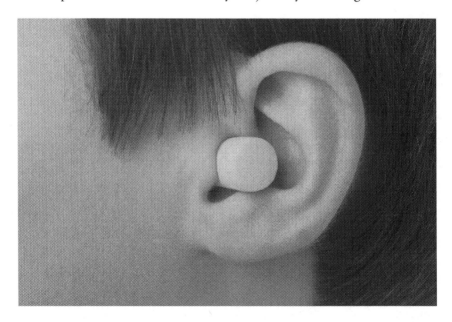

## Stressful Sounds

Okay when our hearing is not in jeopardy what about our nerves? 59% of people surveyed admit their partners **snore**. Have you ever heard your parents fighting or a couple yell thru a hotel wall? Have you witnessed a sports team brawl, heard a loud explosion, or heard someone wail at the loss of someone they love? Have you heard a **baby cry,** screaming in the night, or a child holler to the high heavens because they can't have chocolate ice cream?

Have **hiccups** annoyed you, a **burp** embarrass you, or the other baby sounds that comes from too much beans and rice? Do you know someone who groans with aches and pains, or listened to a deafening gunshot on the city streets, or on a television show?

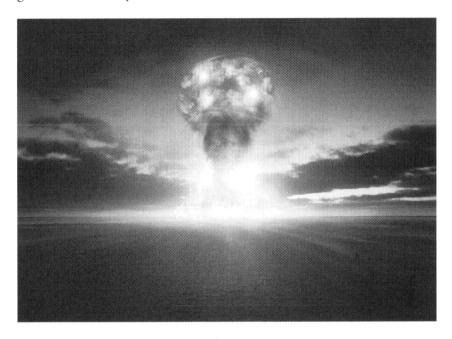

Does the intense memory of **war** play in your brain filling your head with a cacophony of sounds night after night?

Has a hurricane torn off your roof or torn down your barn, or have you heard the sheep or chicken let out an ear-piercing cry when a wolf is in sight? Have you heard a horse "neigh," or a plane crash, or a fire sweep thru a house, or wooded area with a crackling snap and a roaring intensity of destruction and terror?

Have you heard a car crash, a pot or pan clank, or a glass shatter with shrill delight? Not all sounds have to be at decibels to destroy the eardrums some manage to destroy our hearts and our lives. How can we cope with sounds that tear our world or our serenity apart?

**Sound sensitivities** can induce trauma on our life: memories, screeching, cries, even birds on the windowsill, woodpeckers working diligently against the tree, early morning trash trucks, neighbors yelling, cats in heat, a housemate's TV that's too loud, memories of war, or even a song that takes us back to a moment in time that our life was moved or touched in some way. How do we block out or deal with sounds that touch our world and our life?

Can you plug your ears? Go ahead and try it. Cup your hands over your ears and listen to that sound? Is it familiar? Yes that's the heartbeat of the mother, that womb sound — the cacophony of inner peace and tranquility, which lies within us all. You can train yourself to hear that inner sound. In only 3 – 5 minutes a day, you can become a master at: blocking sound, sound ease, sounds control and sound magic. Would you like to be able to stand in the center of Grand Central Station and hear absolute silence? With a little practice you can feel peace; you can master and capture the inner beauty of nothingness, stillness and complete happiness as a daily part of your life.

You will find practicing **sound meditations** are very relaxing. You can hear the warm blood flowing through your body and you can listen to the beating of your heart. You can tap into the electrical output of your brain, and the music of spheres dancing thru you in harmony and delight. The music of the octaves of heaven lies in each and every one of us. You need only quiet the mind and listen. It will soothe you, open you and allow you to live in a peaceful tranquil space where noise is not in your circle but simply lives in the outside, outside world.

> *"Always Listen To Your Heart*
> *Because, even though it's on the left side it's always right."*

Have you ever stood under a waterfall? Lovely isn't it? Tropical, enchanted, the wondrous paradise part of what we love is the whooshing sound of the water over our: heads, ears, and flowing vigorously over our body — swaddling us in perfection, and drenching us in the sweet essence of life, power, glory and the all that is.

We are cleansed of our sins, our problems, our woes, our pains and anything that separates us from nature and from ourselves.

Since we can't all go to the Caribbean today or to Hawaii's sandy shores, your shower has the same power and it awaits you. Just running the water over your head is very relaxing and it's an easy key and tool to cancel unwanted sound, even those that are clanking around in our heads. **Showers** are the gifts of the modern world.

Another glorious stress-saving technique is a **fan**. That's right! No: not the one that has a camera, and is following you around with an autograph book, and a pen. **We're talking about an electrical fan that you can buy in any hardware or department store.** It doesn't have to be new-fangled, have loads of settings or even cost a fortune. It can be a simple, easy, honest to goodness fan. When you are having trouble sleeping, just get a fan and turn it away from you so the air is not blowing directly on your body and let the sound slowly lull you to sleep.

That whoosh from the Mother's womb is what we hear as we listen to the fan… within minutes you'll be off in dreamland: safe, secure, content, and at peace. Your emotions are ready for wondrous and beautiful dreams, a restful sleep and a night that feels like your childhood; where you can snuggle down and know that everything is all right and it is. So sleep easy with **one single fan**.

Others choose a **white noise machine**. This is also a fine choice and readily available in today's market. You can even purchase one online and what a tremendous gift you have just given to yourself. A white noise machine can block out: cars outside, rustling noises, trees swooshing in the wind, neighbors coming and going, street sweepers, or any outside world interference. The white noise machine works like an internal engine in your brain and soon you will be drifting off without a care in the world. This is always an excellent solution not to mention a very generous gift to those you love.

## CHAPTER 10

# THE EYES ARE OUR GATEWAYS TO HAPPINESS

Did you know that your sight could be affected by Stress?

Have you ever heard someone say; I'm so
angry I can't even see straight?

Or heard someone share; that they're seeing red?

Stress affects our eyes.

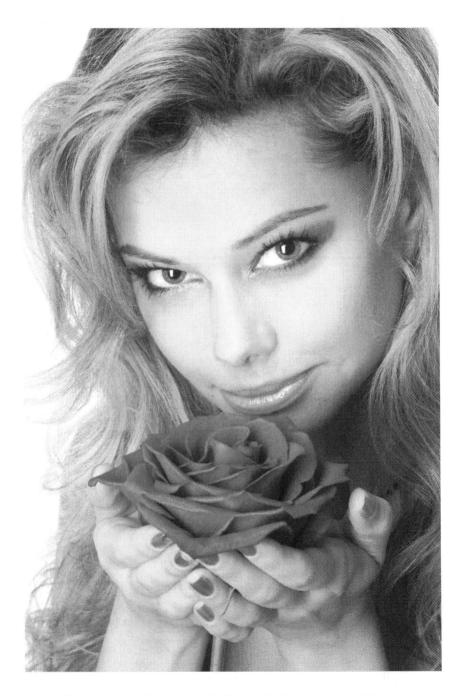

*"Everything that is made beautiful and fair and lovely*
*Is, made for the eye of one who sees." -- Rumi*

Our eyes are hungry and they crave nutrients the same way our bodies do. They thrive when we give them delightful herbs that nourish our eyes, and free them from the bondage of overuse and neglect. The **Bilberry Herb** is comforting and delightful to the eye. This satisfies the eyes hunger for nourishment and love.

The Air Force found **Vitamin A** helpful in sharpening the vision and peripheral sight.

We bath our bodies and luxuriate in various washes and products to make us feel smooth, silky and clean. Our eyes can be bathed as well. **Eyebright** is a wonderfully, successful **eyewash** available on the market today!

**E-W (Eye Wash)** can be taken internally, and can be easily found at your local health food store. Or you can make **a tea with just 3 capsules per cup**. Let the tea steep for 20 minutes and then, for decadence, put it in a jar and leave it in the refrigerator overnight.

This makes a fabulous eye wash in the morning, and the healing properties go back thru the history of time. Use this **highbred eyewash** when it's cooled to cleanse the eye. When you remove it from the fridge don't agitate it, let the sediment settle, as it will. Use your eyecup to rinse your eyes, and this one lot will last for 3 to 4 washes for both eyes during the day. The original eyewash formula was developed by Dr. John Christopher and E-W follows many of the core ingredients we use today. This is a fantastic cure and reliever for vascular degeneration, sties, glaucoma, cataracts and almost any eye condition imaginable.

**Warm compresses**, **hot washcloths** or even **warm tea bags** are wonderful solutions to relaxing and indulging our eyes and our senses.

*"Maybe that's what life is... a wink of the eye and winking stars."*

*-- Jack Kerouac*

**Winking and Blinking**: Okay who hasn't seduced another soul by just blinking, winking or batting their eye? The brain is like a camera blinking so often. It's just like our breathing it can be conscious or unconscious. We can choose to take a deep relaxing breath or we can just breathe as we do, second to second to stay alive, function and continue on this golden path we call life. We can choose to blink for effect, to say; a-okay or to lure someone in, however our eyes will naturally blink whether we'd like them to or not. A blink, cleanses the eye, lubricates your camera and your lens to the world.

## *"In a dark time, the eye begins to see."*

### *– Cavett Robert*

Have you seen the commercials for **dry eyes**? They say it's a disease. When your eyes are dried out, you can get cataracts. Now who wouldn't want to prevent that?

Have you ever wanted to snuggle with your love one by the warm hearth of a fireplace on a romantic night? Does the bonfire at the beach or roasting marshmallows delight you? Did you know that fire quickly stresses and dries out your eyes? So what can you do about it so you can enjoy those romantic and intoxicating nights?

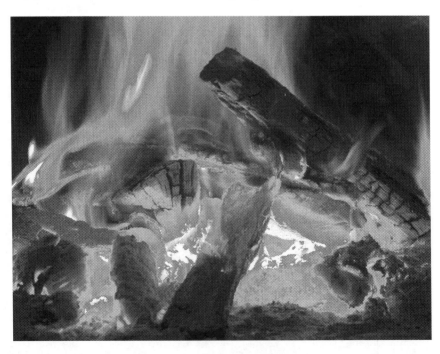

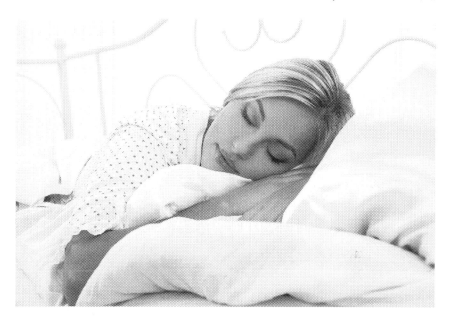

Plain, organic, cold pressed **Flax Oil** works wonders. Let it settle a little in the refrigerator (don't shake it). Be patient, **it has to be cold pressed, not chemically pressed.** When you go to bed, fill an eyedropper with the refrigerated Flax Oil, and gently carry that dropper with you to bed. Lay it on the bedside table, it is there to help you heal, rejuvenate, repair and nourish you as you sleep. When you're ready to turn out the light and slumber off to beautiful dreams, place one drop of the Flax Oil from the dropper in each eye. Magic will happen and you are well on your way to healthy lubricated eyes.

**"The Health of the eye seems to demand a horizon. We are never too tired as long as we can see far enough."**

**--Ralph Waldo Emerson**

Okay, how many of you spend hours upon hours each day just staring at your computer? The eyes get lazy and the muscles tend to lose their focus, agility, strength, flexibility and power. The easiest solution is to simply **move your monitor**. The monitor should be straight ahead of you or just "slightly" downward. Don't put the computer on your lap!

It's important to **change the focal distance**. Put something right in front of your face. Can you see it? Of course you can. Now immediately shift your focus to the far wall. Great!!! Then look out the window and shift your focus to the distance. Brilliant, you have just exercised your eyes and the benefits will be astounding for years to come.

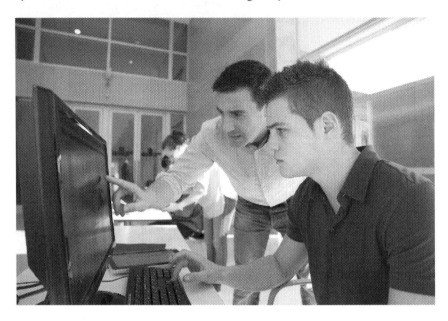

## The Eyes are the Windows to the Soul

Have you ever seen an **Alzheimer's** patient stare? They seem lost and confused, almost not at home inside themselves. And this observation prompts us to remember the saying that, *"The eyes are the windows to the soul."* Protect your eyes; they are the only ones you'll ever have.

We find our memories in using the **movement of our eyes**. It's the movement of the eyes when looking up, straight ahead or looking down, with side to side and up and down; and circular motion. That movement brings up the memory of either the picture of something, the sound of something, or the feeling of something.

Eye exercises that stimulate the **Reticular Formation** throughout the brain help us recall our memories and are great for preventing Alzheimer's:

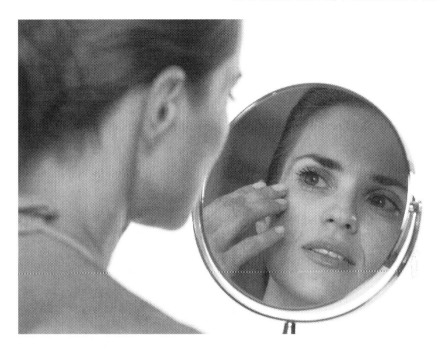

> Look in the mirror and circle your eyes in one direction and then circle in the other direction. This is a great exercise to keep your eyes healthy and the memory strong!

> Now look to the side then up, now the side and down. All of these have phenomenal results in memory and sight capacity. These simple exercises can change your life, the quality of your life, and give you the gift of remembering the life you were here to live.

What happens when your **eyes are strained** from reading, or from scrunching your eyes when you are thinking too hard, or from over-thinking more than you have to – only bad things. Always protect your eyesight! Make sure you have proper lighting. **Sometimes a large magnifying glass can make all the difference.** Once you are older than 40 years, your eyes change their shape and most people require reading glasses.

And those who resist the need for glasses, or a magnifying glass, because of vanity often develop a habit of scrunching their brows to see. And, because of that, lines develop on your face between your eyebrows, and around your eyes. We've all seen people like that. And these lines signal that you, my friend, have been so stressed and now you look 5-10 years older.

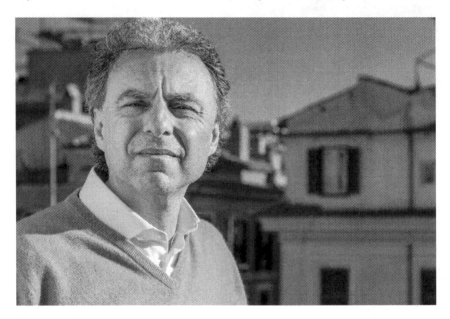

The **Bates Eye Muscle Exercises** can be used to change your focus. You can literally concentrate and focus your eyes.

Also not allowing the light to enter into the eyes can be helpful. You can feel that when you squint. You can practice a very effective technique called **palming**.

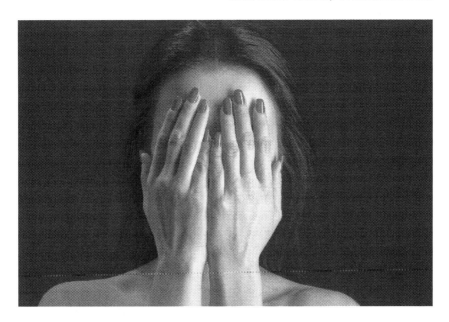

**Palming:** You rub your hands strongly and vigorously together and then cup the eyes and stare in the blackness. This warmth, energy, and darkness combo proves to be a very effective and useful technique for relaxing the muscles and the eyes.

*"Never bend your head. Always hold it high.*
*Look the world straight in the eye."*

*-- Helen Keller*

**Imagine a hero like Helen Keller making such an insightful comment.** Your eyes and your body have the capacity to tolerate pain, especially when you know it's only for limited time frame. A shot at the doctor's office: tying up your ice skates, fitting into a wedding corset or gown, losing one's virginity, running the last leg in a marathon or race, having our ears pierced, tattoos, setting a broken limb, finger or toe, even chemotherapy is endured when we know it is for only a set limit of time. So what about three seconds? What if in a mere three seconds you could relieve stress? What if, that little bit of pressure you feel, is the answer, the solution and the doorway to the other side of success? What if the tools you needed were just your own two hands? That's right the power to success is right in front of you this very instant. Take your hands and **press deep** into your eyes. Hold really tight and penetrate and push a little harder; **do not push or press so hard as to HURT YOURSELF**. See the colors dance and change right before your eyes. Watch as the colors brighten and move, as if alive. Those colors that you see and that tinge that you feel, is the awakening, the recovery, the blossoming and the **opening of your vision** — both internal and external — like never before.

> *"Sometimes the heart sees what is invisible to the eye."*
> *– H. Jackson Brown, Jr.*

**Eye masks** can be quite a treat for sore, tired and restless eyes. **Ice packs** and **ice masks** can do wonders for puffy, swollen eyes. So the next time you're crying thru your favorite movie, or staying up all night studying for an exam, or the effects of sunburn on your eyes from a boat ride. **This is the solution for you!**

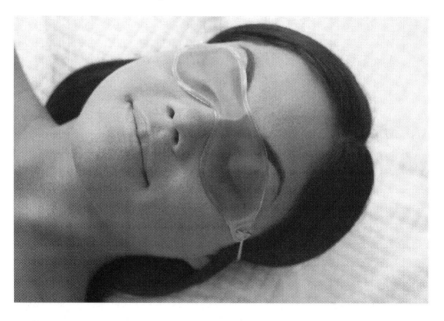

Sunbeams of Life

# CHAPTER 11

# SPEAK NO EVIL

In 30 seconds, you can create enough chemical imbalances to cripple you for life, render you insane, or kill you! **THINK ABOUT THIS before you react, and get upset, or blow your top!**

Our **negative attitudes** and **emotions** cause muscle constriction, and slow down the very life-giving fluids flowing through our bodies! **It is this constriction** that causes the stress response and accelerated aging – and not the emotion itself.

Our **anger** can cause stress rates that actually jump off the charts.

Have you ever said something and regretted what you said — after you said it — or have you ever not said something, and later regretted holding your tongue, your thoughts or your heart?

It is the same exercise with **passion**. Anger is simply the life lesson of passion. Anger unconsciously draws in passion and it teaches us something profound. After all, you can't be angry about something that you don't care about. Whether kicked, battered, beaten or emotionally traumatized, anger comes in an instant and it leaves in the proverbial 5 minutes. It develops passion and it teaches us to care about something, to care about anything; it helps us to care.

Every emotion on the human spectrum is a seesaw. On one side the raw feeling and on the other side a life lesson to be cherished and adored. We've all played that emotional game of the ups and downs ever since the second we were born. We screamed and cried and then cooed peacefully in an instant. By now we have mastered this process.

Passion is a good thing; it is just that anger is a painful way of learning it.

> *"Anger is our natural defense against pain.*
> *So when you say, 'I hate you,"*
> *It really means: You Hurt ME.*

# You will not be punished for your anger, You will be punished by your anger.

If anger is an **emotional exercise,** then what is **resentment**? Do you ever remember being spanked or being yelled at in front of others? Did someone put you down or make fun of you? Were you ever bullied or picked on?

Did someone take something that you thought belonged to you? Were you tripped along your path, stopped from living your dreams, or not given the proper tools to live the life you wanted to live? Have you ever muttered or whispered, even silently in your own heart; *"I'll get even with you, even if it takes my whole life. I'll get even! Just you wait!"* Do you remember what happened the next week? We focused, we concentrated, and we even obsessed on almost nothing else except, getting even!

Resentment is the unconscious exercise that teaches us **the tools of focus, concentration, how to stay on point, how to aim for a target or a goal** and the great lesson of **forgiveness**. Focus, concentration, and being on point are great things to learn; resentment is just a very painful way to learn it.

Imagine a window and a man is looking out enjoying the morning sun. Across the street there is an open window. He can see a man in the house across the street sitting quietly with his hands immobile in his lap, and there is another man in conversation with him, raging and pacing like a Bengal tiger. He is screaming at the top of his lungs and throwing things about.

To the spectator, the one man is crazy and infuriated, and the other man is simply meek, and the victim of his insanity. The truth is; they both might be feeling the same intensity of **rage** inside. The only difference is in what they do with their bodies. That's the difference between the **animal man** and the **spiritual man**. **Animal man always constricts his body while spiritual man chooses to relax his body; yet they both feel the same.**

Is it possible to relax when anger overtakes us? Yes, you cannot stop a feeling; you can only change how you relate to it. Have you ever seen someone angry who grits their teeth or holds their breath? Often when we're angry, we'll squeeze our butt cheeks or clench our fists. Sometimes when we feel provoked or kicked into an emotion like anger, there are ways to balance our anger and volatility by choosing the spiritual man over the animal man.

How you ask? By choosing what to do with our bodies, to relax our jaw or fists, and unclench our butt cheeks. It is a healthier way to lead our lives. Even **journaling** or **drawing a picture** can take your focus to a new, and healthier space by developing the **small motor skills** and muscles, and it can immediately change how your mind is working. To use the small motor skills while writing, you must think while acting.

**Exercise** and **sex**, taking **walks,** and **being in nature while playing** develop the **large motor skills** and **muscles.** They teach us how to use our bodies so that we have choice. Here we have the opportunity to handle things very differently simply by choosing **how** we use our bodies in connection with our stress. Have you ever wish you handled a situation in a very different way? These tools are available to you; it's a simple choice and **divine living** can be yours.

We can choose constriction or relaxation? You have **the choice.**

Every negative emotion teaches us a powerful lesson. **Depression** is rabid in today's society. The outside circumstances seem to tackle our worlds with such force, fervor, and determination, that many people find it hard to get back up. Depression teaches us the deep lesson of **introspection**. While studying in India, we learned that there is no word for depression; it is an innate knowing and inner sense. The blanket of emotions one is saddled with is simply **unguided introspection.**

Practices like meditating, yoga, and quieting the mind allow you to peacefully go inward. They allow you to discover the proper tools to calmly and insightfully see the messages, lessons; and truths that come with our emotions, and our passions in our lives. Introspection is a good thing; it's just that depression is a painful way of learning it.

**Fear** is a great **imagination** builder. Don't you remember when there were monsters in your closet, or the "boogie man" was coming to get you or hiding under your bed? Fear allows us to **expand our mind and consciousness** to all the realms of possibilities and scenarios of (what can happen), and we can make it as big and as vivid, and as detailed as we like.

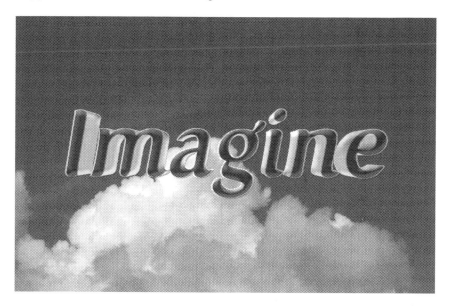

Our stories — whether they are 'ghost stories by a campfire' or the ones we tell ourselves that are rattling in our head — can create a phenomenal realm of fantasy, exploration, adventures; journeying, and imagination beyond our wildest dreams. Imagination is a good thing; however, it's just that fear is a painful way of learning it. Indeed, positive imagining is the birthplace of great ideas.

**Everything teaches us something** — the secret is to learn what the lesson is. Then the counseling changes in our lives because we never thought of the lessons before. Easy options like getting our **biorhythm**

chart can clarify our physical, emotional and mental rhythms. You can go online and "Google" biorhythms and then just put in your birthday. It's an easy exercise to do, and the results you will find will astound you.

We all have a choice. You can choose what you're having for dinner tonight and you can choose your **emotional pattern** in life. Ask yourself, *"What choice do I have with my body?"* Imagine an actor who plays a part, and chooses to let that rollercoaster of emotion bubble up and percolate with precision, skill and mastery. Or picture an athlete who has the flu yet, decides to play anyway and wins the game for the team, overriding his physical urge to go back to bed.

Or the injured dancer who is the lead in the ballet – the audience has been seated, and there is excitement and anticipation to see the performance begin. That dancer takes a breath and steps on stage, compartmentalizing their pain, injury and trauma. We all have the skills to step gracefully onto the stages of our lives. This book teaches you how to live spiritually and harmoniously within your own realm of consciousness and magic.

**Remember we rule our emotions, and our emotions do not rule us.**

**You have choice — choose wisely and happiness can be yours.**

**Another way of expressing this is:**

**You must become master of your mind,**

**And not let your mind master you.**

**A real friend is kind, but straightforward,**

**Caring but forceful, understanding but honest.**

**You can always count on them to tell you the truth.**

# CHAPTER 12

# WAYS TO DEAL WITH STRESS

You can use a number of methods to cope with stress, experiment to find the ones that work best for you. You may want to check with your doctor before using these techniques.

**Muscle tension and release**: Lie down in a quiet room. Take a slow, deep breath. As you breathe in, tense a particular muscle or group of muscles. For example: you can squeeze your eyes shut, frown, clench your teeth, make a fist, or stiffen your arms or legs. Hold your breath and keep your muscles tense for a second or two. Then breathe out, release the tension, and let your body relax **completely**. Repeat the process with another muscle or muscle group.

You also can try a variation of this method, called "**progressive relaxation**." Start with the toes of one foot and, working upward, progressively tense and relax all the muscles of one leg. Next, do the same with the other leg. Then tense and relax the rest of the muscle groups in your body, including those in your scalp. Remember to hold your breath while tensing your muscles and to breathe out when releasing the tension.

**Rhythmic breathing**: Get into a comfortable position and relax all your muscles. When you keep your eyes open, focus on a distant object. When you close your eyes, imagine a peaceful scene or simply clear your mind and focus on the colors you see, while you control your breathing. Breathe in and out slowly and comfortably through your nose. If you like, you might keep the rhythm steady by saying to yourself, "In, one two — Out, one two." Feel yourself **relax and go limp** each time you breathe out.

You can do this technique for just a few seconds or for up to 10 minutes. You can gently slow your rhythmic breathing down by counting slowly and silently to three. Breathe gently and relax.

**Biofeedback**: With training in biofeedback, you can control body functions such as heart rate, blood pressure, and muscle tension. A machine will sense when your body shows signs of tension and will let you know in some way such as making a sound or flashing a light. The machine will also give you feedback when you relax your body. Eventually, you will be able to control your relaxation responses without having to depend on feedback from the machine. Your doctor or nurse can refer you to a biofeedback trainer in your local area.

**Imagery**: Imagery is a way of daydreaming that uses all your senses. It usually is done with your eyes closed. To begin, breathe slowly and feel yourself relax. Imagine a ball of healing energy — perhaps a white light, forming somewhere in your body. When you can "see" the ball of energy, imagine that as you breathe in. You can blow the ball to any part of the body where you feel pain, tension, or discomfort. When you breathe out, picture the air moving the ball away from your body, taking with it any painful or uncomfortable feelings. (Be sure to breathe naturally; there's no need to blow.) Continue to picture the ball moving toward you and away from you, each time you breathe in and out. You may see the ball getting bigger and bigger as it takes away more and more of your tension and discomfort.

To end the imagery, just count slowly to three; breathe in deeply, gently open your eyes, and say to yourself out loud, **"I feel alert and relaxed."**

**Visualization**: Visualization is a method that is similar to imagery. With visualization, you create an inner picture that represents your fight against stress, illness, pain or any disease, discomfort or unhappiness. Some people getting chemotherapy use images of rockets blasting away their cancer cells, or of knights in armor battling their cancer cells. Others create an image of their white blood cells or their drugs attacking the cancer cells. You can use similar imagery to fight any battle or to overcome any pain, stress, wall or hurdle in your way. You have the inner power, ability and strength to heal your body, mind, soul and heart.

**Hypnosis**: Hypnosis puts you in a trance-like state that can help reduce discomfort and anxiety. A qualified person can hypnotize you; or you can learn how to hypnotize yourself. Whenever you are interested in learning more, ask your doctor or nurse to refer you to someone highly trained in this effective technique.

**Distraction**: You can use distraction at any time by choosing an activity to take your mind off your worries, discomforts or fears: watching TV, listening to the radio, reading, going to the movies, or working with your hands — (small motor skills) — by doing needlework or puzzles, building models, or painting. You may be surprised how comfortable you are and how quickly the time passes.

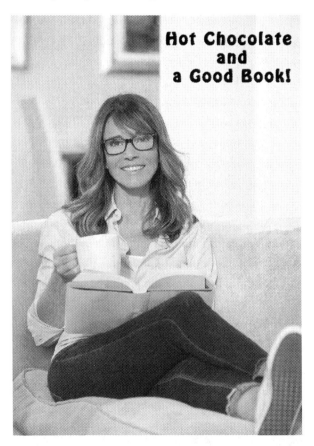

Hot Chocolate and a Good Book!

## CHAPTER 13

# WATER IS NATURE'S QUINTESSENTIAL ANSWER

## Moses: Then the sea parted!

## How powerful is our image of water?

### *"Water is the Driving Force of All Nature."*

### *-- Leonardo da Vinci*

We are naturally drawn to dancing waterfalls, placid lakes, rolling rivers, powerful oceans and the invitation of the sea. So then why do we have so much trouble consuming water in our daily lives? Natural drinking water is the most precious and blessed gift we have.

Today's commercials have sold us on the popularity of sugared soft drinks, liquor, artificially-flavored *Slurpees*; and also powdered, flavored and processed milk.

When the world was created, you remember, way before the Coke and Pepsi industry; we were given to this planet, the gift of water.

**Water** used to be free; it flowed effortlessly over our lands and our shores. We built homes where water poured out of the faucets, and it danced though our hoses with gregarious delight...

Water is the essence and the symbol of life. We were born, protected and nurtured in our own cocoon and canopy of water.

Our bodies need, long for, want and desire water.

Water actually helps with **weight loss.** You don't have to give up that pizza just drink some water!

### Benefits of drinking 1-2 liters a day:

It powers your workouts. Have 2 glasses before your workouts. And every thirty minutes exercising, drink one more glass of water.

Water also speeds up your fat metabolism. Sweating increases one's caloric burning. A fancy word for this is "Thermogenesis."

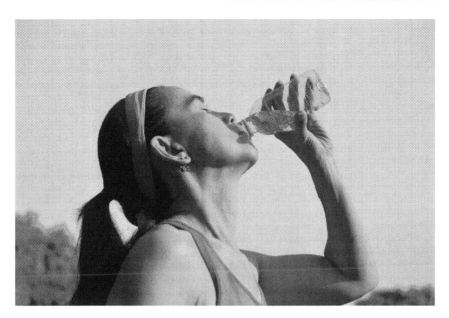

Water fiercely helps in the **prevention of stress and heart attacks**.

Did you know that simply drinking a glass of water 45 minutes before each meal can change your life?

We eagerly recommend that you drink a glass of water as a compliment to your meal. Water has the power to effectively aid in the digestion and absorption of vital minerals and essential nutrients for your body to use, just make sure that it is room temperature.

Ice is not necessary… water is perfect just the way it is. Our ancestors in the deserts, and our relatives who rode across the Wild, Wild West to: settle people into communities and a free, wondrous life that did not have ice cubes, automatic icemakers, or even ice trays to cube their water with.

For cold water we had snow, icicles and sleet. Natural water at natural room temperature is what our body craves, yearns for and desires.

**"We forget that the water cycle and the life cycles are one."**

-- *Jacques Yves Cousteau*

*"An entire sea of water can't sink a ship unless it gets inside. Similarly, the negativity of the world can't put you down, unless you allow it inside your heart and mind."*

— **Unknown**

*"The water in a vessel is sparkling; the water in the sea is dark. The small truth has words that are clear; the great truth has great silence."*

— *Rabindranath Tagore*

**The first thing in the morning our body needs is water.** Have you ever seen someone throw a glass or a bucket of ice on someone to wake them up? Yes it works, only **wouldn't you rather drink a glass of thirst quenching water to start your day with energy, vitality and optimal health?**

*"To live is the rarest thing in the world. Most people exist, that is all."*

— *Oscar Wilde*

*"Thousands have lived without love, not one without water."*

— *W. H. Auden*

*Unlike a drop of water, which loses its identity when it joins the ocean, man does not lose his being in the society in which he lives. Man's life is independent. He is born not for the development of the society alone, but for the development of his self.*

— **B. R. Ambedkar**

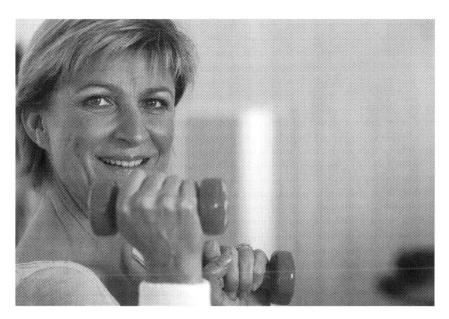

*"I have dreamed in my life, dreams that have stayed with me after, and changed my ideas. They have gone through me, like wine through water, and altered the color of my mind."*

*--Emily Bronte*

Bedtime is the perfect time to give thanks for your day. You may have evening rituals like saying your prayers, setting out your clothes for the next day, answering e-mails, reading a book; turning on the TV, or kissing your loved one goodnight. However, before you do something, what your body is looking for is a glass of water. Statistics prove that just one glass of room temperature water before going to bed can assist in a deep and **restful sleep**. That water will quickly **lubricate your joints**, **hydrate your organs and muscles** and actually fend off **heart attacks** and **strokes**.

That's right, most heart attacks and strokes actually happen first thing in the morning, after the body has been compromised by lack of hydration. When you wake up, the system rebels and it shuts down.

Imagine if your heart attack or stroke can be prevented or, on the other hand, could have been prevented by simply drinking a glass of water before you head off to sleep. That's reason enough to hydrate your body before you slumber.

*"For true love is inexhaustible; the more you give, the more you have. And if you go to draw at the fountainhead; the more water you draw; the more abundant is its flow."*

*--Antoine de Saint-Exupery*

Our life flows effortlessly through the days, weeks and years. That flow of water through the day gives you energy, and feeds your mind, body and soul. During the day, optimally 2 hours after a meal, you will find your body has worked hard to digest and process your food. **Water at this time is perfect** as it helps to thin out what's in your stomach, and allows for better movement, as everything travels through the entire intestinal tract. Now you will easily absorb the nutrients you just ate.

Rewarding your body with a glass of water 2 hours after a delectable meal provides **instant health** and **energy** and it opens the doorways for a glorious day of stress free living?

*"Take a course in good water and air; and in the eternal youth of Nature you may renew your own. Go quietly, alone; no harm will befall you."*

*–John Muir*

*"Anyone who has never made a mistake has never tried anything new."*

*–Albert Einstein*

*"We do no great things, only small things with great love."*

*—Mother Teresa*

# CHAPTER 14

# WE HAVE SEEN ENOUGH

*"If we doctors threw all our medicines into the sea, it would be that much better for our patients and that much worse for the fishes."*

*-- Supreme Court Justice Oliver Wendell Holmes, MD*

We have seen the foolishness of the conventional wisdom pertaining to disease care. We have seen hospitals feed white bread to patients with bowel cancer and "Jell-O" to patients with leukemia. We have seen schools feed bright red "Slush Puppies" for lunch to 7-year-olds who vomit up a desk-top full of red crud afterwards. We have seen those same children line up later at the school nurse's office for hyperactivity drugs.

We have seen patients in hospitals who were allowed to go two weeks without a bowel movement, and told it was OK. We have seen patients who were told that they had six months to live, when they might actually have lived sixty months. We have seen people recover from serious illness, only to have their physician berate them for having used natural healing methods to do so. We have seen infants spit up formula while their mothers were advised not to breast-feed. We have seen better ingredients in dog food than in the average school or hospital lunch.

**We have seen enough!**

One of the most dangerous weapons in the world is the table fork. Don't bother looking in the history books for what has killed the most Americans. Look, instead, at your breakfast, lunch, and dinner table. There's an old saying: *"One fourth of what you eat keeps you alive. The other three fourths keep your doctor alive."* We eat too much of the wrong things and not enough of the right things. Scientific research continually indicates rampant nationwide vitamin and mineral deficiencies. **We spend over one trillion dollars each year on disease care in America — and almost nothing on prevention.** Is it any surprise that doctors consistently place among the very highest per capita income levels in the country?

*"And we have made of ourselves living cesspools, and driven doctors to invent names for our diseases."*

**-- *Plato***

About 10 million U.S. soldiers were killed in World War I, having faced an enemy armed with machine guns and bayonets. There were nearly a million casualties at the Somme and another million at Verdun, just to mention two of the battles. The horrific slaughter of this war went on for four years. **Yet, in just the two years following the war, over 20 million people died from influenza. That is more than twice as many deaths from the flu in one-half the time it took armed opposition.**

During the American Civil War, in which nearly two thirds of a million soldiers died, **three times as many soldiers died from disease as from battle**. Today, **alcohol and tobacco kill nearly as many Americans in one year as the entire Civil War did in four.** Today, we lose more than a million Americans each year to cancer and heart disease. These are staggering statistics.

So always remember **that disease is the real enemy and most of the time, it is self-induced.**

Results are all that matter. Alternative medicine works. The natural treatment of illness can be accomplished safely, inexpensively and effectively. We've all been taught that anything that is safe and inexpensive cannot possibly be truly effective against "real diseases." It is time to rethink that — to experiment and see for yourself what works.

Our work does not involve prescription. It involves description and information. It is important for us to be free to utilize any reasonable health care approach that we deem viable. To make an educated decision, we need more education.

Natural healing is not about avoiding doctors. It is about not needing to go to doctors in the first place. To follow a proper lifestyle is to prevent disease. A dentist is not upset when you are cavity-free. A doctor should not be upset when you are healthy, yet the medical system thrives on sickness and disease. The whole idea is to be healthy.

The first step must be in the desire to want to be healthy. **The old Chinese saying is "When you are sick of sickness, you are no longer sick." That is the start to wellness.**

The second step is to do something to **improve your health**. Each of us is ultimately responsible for our own wellness; and we should leave no stone unturned in our search for how to have better health. *You get out of your body what you put into it*. Your body will respond to your efforts to improve your health. It is up to you, and no one else; you are responsible for how you live. The only thing that gets rid of ignorance about what your body needs, and how to live healthfully is by knowledge, and that takes effort; effort you get to joyfully put in.

*"Each treatment regimen I utilize in my practice is not exclusively mine. I do not stay up late at night making all this up. These ideas are not original. They are generally not new, either. Rather, they are a culmination, a hybrid, of the work of all the pioneers in the alternative health field. This is the foundation upon which I continue to build. I have collected, and continue to collect, the safest and most effective healing approaches that I can find from physicians worldwide. I hope you find them to be as helpful as they have been for my patients and my family."*

*– Dr. Ben-Joseph*

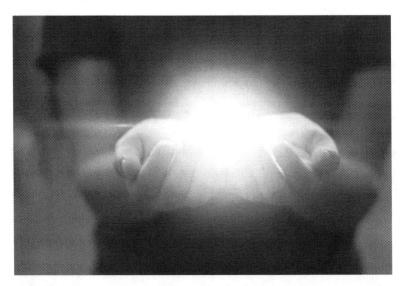

# CHAPTER 15

# 10 TIPS FOR HEALTHY EATING

Experts agree the key to healthy eating is the time-tested advice of **balance**, **variety** and **moderation**.

Eating a wide variety of colorful foods will add **fuel, strength and vitality** to your world, especially **foods rich in nutrients** and **essential vitamins and minerals**.

These **10 tips** can help you live a healthier, stronger, and more vibrant life; while still enjoying your favorite foods and lifestyle.

*1. Eat a variety of nutrient-rich, colorful foods.* More than **91** different **nutrients** are needed for our good **health, wellness, longevity, brain function** and optimum **mobility and movement**. We need 12 amino acids (9 essential and 3 mostly essential), 16 vitamins, 3 fatty acids, and 60 minerals. **No single food is the super hero.** Each individual nutrient plays a significant part in the healthy and happier version of you!

Your daily food selection needs to include whole-grain non-GMO products (read labels – some breads may contain high levels of GMO products and nasty chemicals and don't forget – lots of sugar). When you're going to eat healthy, do it right and choose high-quality colorful, fresh food whenever possible. Your daily intake needs to include fruits, vegetables, raw dairy products (or none when allergic); grass fed meats, hormone and antibiotic free poultry, and wild cold-water fish, and other high protein foods like raw seeds and nuts or omega 3 eggs.

How much you need to eat depends on your calorie needs.

*2. Enjoy plenty of* **fruits, vegetables and non-GMO whole grains.** 2-4 servings of fruit can kick start your day and offer a healthy alternative or snack between any meals. 3-5 servings of vegetables are imperative for a healthy lifestyle. 6-11 servings from the bread, rice, cereal and pasta group are **highly effective fiber for great eliminations** (make sure all grains are non-GMO). Also, including 3 servings from the whole grains category can literally change your life in the morning, as you can finally do something sitting on the throne. You can always look through cookbooks, or go online for tasty ways to prepare unfamiliar foods. You'll be surprised at what you can create in a brief amount of time. From mere seconds to mere minutes fantastic, delectable and scrumptious delights can be feeding your body, mind, spirit and soul. You can use and the Nutrition Facts panel on food labels and the Food Guide Pyramid as handy references.

Sample Label for
Macaroni and Cheese

**Start Here**

**Nutrition Facts**
Serving Size 1 cup (228g)
Servings Per Container 2

| Amount Per Serving | |
|---|---|
| Calories 250 | Calories from Fat 110 |

| | % Daily Value* |
|---|---|
| Total Fat 12g | 18% |
| Saturated Fat 3g | 15% |
| *Trans* Fat 1.5g | |
| Cholesterol 30mg | 10% |
| Sodium 470mg | 20% |
| Total Carbohydrate 31g | 10% |
| Dietary Fiber 0g | 0% |
| Sugars 5g | |
| Protein 5g | |

| | |
|---|---|
| Vitamin A | 4% |
| Vitamin C | 2% |
| Calcium | 20% |
| Iron | 4% |

* Percent Daily Values are based on a 2,000 calorie diet. Your Daily Values may be higher or lower depending on your calorie needs:

| | Calories: | 2,000 | 2,500 |
|---|---|---|---|
| Total Fat | Less than | 65g | 80g |
| Sat Fat | Less than | 20g | 25g |
| Cholesterol | Less than | 300mg | 300mg |
| Sodium | Less than | 2,400mg | 2,400mg |
| Total Carbohydrate | | 300g | 375g |
| Dietary Fiber | | 25g | 30g |

**Limit these Nutrients**

**Get Enough of these Nutrients**

**Footnote**

**Quick Guide to % DV**
5% or less is low
20% or more is high

**New Nutritional Label**

*3*. **Maintain a healthy weight.** The weight that's right for you depends on many factors including your sex, height, age and heredity. Excess **body fat** increases your chances for **high blood pressure, heart disease, stroke, diabetes**, some types of **cancer** and other illnesses. Also, being too thin can increase your risk for **osteoporosis**, and for women, it can also affect **menstrual irregularities** and other health problems. When you're constantly losing and regaining weight, a Traditional Naturopath can help you in developing sensible eating habits for successful weight management. **Regular exercise** is also important to maintaining a healthy weight.

4. **Eat moderate portions**. When you keep portion sizes reasonable, it's easier to eat the foods you desire and to stay healthy. Did you know the recommended serving of cooked meat is 3 ounces, similar to the size of a deck of playing cards? A medium piece of fruit is considered 1 serving and a cup of pasta equals 2 servings. A pint of ice cream contains 4 servings. Referring to the **Food Guide Pyramid** is always an excellent source for information on recommended serving portions and sizes.

5. **Eat regular meals**. Skipping meals can lead to out-of-control hunger, often resulting in **overeating or binging**. When you're very hungry, it's also tempting to forget about your good nutrition and a healthy diet and way of life and grab anything that looks like food and just start stuffing your face. You might even find yourself grabbing that sandwich right out of that kids hand and stuffing it into your mouth before you even know it. Snacking between meals can help your hunger, remember **a snack is a small portion of energy and fuel** you can save your entrees for your mealtime.

6. **Reduce; don't eliminate certain foods**. Most people eat for pleasure as well as nutrition. When your favorite foods are junk and high in fat, salt or sugar, the key is moderating how much of these foods you eat and how often you'll eat them. Remember moderation in all things including **moderation**.

Identify major sources of these negative ingredients in your diet and make any necessary changes so that you only eat them once in a while. Adults who eat high-fat processed, chemical-infused meats or hormone antibiotic pus-loaded whole-milk dairy products from regular poorly fed cows and not from pure grass fed cows, at meals are probably consuming too much toxic chemicals. Fat is a great storage container for all of the garbage your body can't get rid of. Learn how to read and use the Nutrition Facts panel on the food label to help balance your choices and know what you are eating.

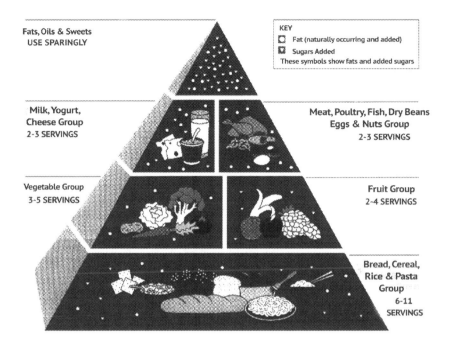

When you love fried chicken, pizza or any junk food, you don't have to give it up, just use your common sense and eat it less often. Be aware of its contents and effects on the body, your energy level and overall system and functionality. This varies for every individual. **When dining out, share the desert with a friend; ask for a take-home bag or a smaller portion**.

*7.* **Balance your food choices over time.** Not every food has to be "perfect." When eating a food high in fat, salt or sugar and chemicals, select other foods that are low in these ingredients. **Whenever you miss out on any food group one day, make up for it the next day.** When you **vary your food** choices over several days, you will notice that most foods will fit together into a healthy pattern.

*8.* **Know your diet pitfalls**. To improve your eating habits, you first have to know what's not working. Write down everything you eat for three days. Then check your list according to the rest of these tips. Do you add a lot of regular hormone butter instead of grass-fed butter. How about creamy milk sauces on GMO pasta or salad dressings with omega

6 oils instead of **omega 3 oils**? Rather than eliminating these foods, just change the ingredients to the healthy one and enjoy. Are you getting enough fruits and vegetables? If not, you may be missing out on vital nutrients so consider a **high-grade vitamin supplement like Prime Longevity – available at primelongevity.com.**

*9.* **Make changes gradually.** Just as there are no single all-in-one "super foods" or easy answers to a healthy diet, don't expect to totally revamp your eating habits overnight. **Changing too much, too fast can get in the way of success**. Begin to remedy excesses or deficiencies, with modest changes that can add up to positive, lifelong eating habit.

*10. Remember,* **foods are not good or bad**. Select foods based on your total eating patterns, not whether any individual food is "good" or "bad." You don't need to feel guilty when you love foods such as apple pie, potato chips, candy bars or ice cream. Eat them in moderation, and choose other foods to provide the balance and variety that are vital to good health. As you change your diet for the better, your desire for these junk foods will diminish and disappear. And when you do consume them, you will feel the food hangover reactions: sluggish, tired, gassy, bloated and changes in your bowels. You will remember these feelings and that memory helps you to say 'no thank you' to something that you once loved. Feeling well, as you eat well, is better than feeling bad when you eat badly.

# CHAPTER 16

# FOOD FOR THOUGHT GUIDELINES

## 28 Rules: FOOD FOR THOUGHT GUIDELINES
## Healthy Eating and Proper Food Choices

The first, which is food combining, is for **individuals with sensitive digestion**. The more sensitive you are — the more you need to follow the instructions. A few individuals may even disregard the food combining instructions, as they are the ones that can *'eat a rock,'* as the expression goes.

Use your judgment and remember the more digestive issues that you have, the more imperative it is that **you must follow the instructions**.

1.  **FOOD COMBINING**. When you mix vinegar with baking powder, you get bubbles. This is a chemical reaction and it will occur whether you mix it in China, Japan, Paris or New York City. This is the foundation of Food Combining. **Improper food combining can result in abdominal pain, cramping, gas, feeling bloated and indigestion.**

There are many rules on how to combine food properly. Some are more important than others. Attempting to follow all of them may result in frustration and discouragement, or totally giving up and not following any rules. Your diet program and simple food combining rules will help you get healthy and stay healthy. The four listed below are the major rules of food combining that need to be followed for optimal health.

**A. DO NOT combine animal protein with starch**

**B. DO NOT combine acid fruit with starch**

**C. DO NOT combine acid fruit with sweet fruit**

**D. DO NOT combine melons with any other foods**

2.  **ROTATION OF FOODS**. The most common reason people become allergic to foods is that they eat those foods often. Variety is the spice of life. By eating a varied diet, we not only maximize our ability to intake vitamins and minerals, we also avoid the potential

hazard of food allergies, sensitivities and intolerances. There are two methods of food rotation:

➤ For severely sensitive people, it is best to eat all you want of a particular food for one day, and not to repeat that same food for four days.

➤ For less sensitive individuals, consume the food for three or four days in a row, and then go a week without eating that food. This also cuts down on spoilage by consuming all of the remaining leftovers.

3.   ANIMAL PROTEIN. Animal proteins may be eaten on an every-other-day basis. The most important aspect of eating animal products is the beef must come from cows that only eat grass, and chickens that eat a high Omega 3 diet and not an Omega 6 diet.

Chicken, fish and meats need to be baked, broiled or sometimes grilled, though **never fried.** Don't forget, **rotate the type of animal protein you eat to avoid getting and food sensitivity.**

The over consumption of animal protein is one of the major contributors to: **osteoporosis, gout, arthritis, clogged arteries (arterial plaque), hypertension and cancer.**

> A. **Eat one day VEGETARIAN. (The Entire Day)**
>
> B. **Eat one day FISH.        (At Lunch or Dinner)**
>
> C. **Eat one day VEGETARIAN. (The Entire Day)**
>
> D. **Eat one day FOWL-EGGS. (At Lunch or Dinner)**
>
> E. **Eat one day VEGETARIAN. (The Entire Day)**
>
> F. **Eat one day RED MEAT. (At Lunch or Dinner & grass fed)**

4.   PORK OR LARD. **Don't eat pork or lard**. Pork is one of the few animals that pass diseases on to humans. The DNA structure of the pork is so similar to humans that many viruses and disease organisms living in the pork will transfer to humans. Remember swine flu and where it came from.

5.   FISH. **Eat deep-sea, scale fish** only. Fish need to be wild, deep-sea, cold water fish only (e.g. Wild Salmon, Sardines, Herring, and Mackerel.) Avoid eating mollusks and crustacean, or all forms of shellfish and all smooth-skin fish, as they are the scavengers of the ocean bottom, living and eating in the pollution of the sea. **All heavy metals: such as mercury, lead, arsenic, and cadmium, sink to the bottom where these scavengers eat and live out their entire lives.**

6.   BEANS AND LEGUMES. **Soak all beans overnight** before cooking, using only filtered, spring or distilled water. In the morning throw water away, rinse the beans, add fresh clean water, and then cook the beans. This will help to avoid the gas, feeling bloated and indigestion that many people experience when eating beans. **Beans may be combined with grains to make complete proteins (e.g. brown rice and beans, rice and lentils, Asian meals).**

**Remember to avoid eating beans and grains with animal proteins at the same meal for optimal digestion.**

7.   NUTS AND SEEDS. **Nuts and seeds need to be unsalted and raw**. Roasted nuts and seeds loose nutrients in processing and are much more difficult to digest. Soaking nuts and seeds overnight in clean water, like soaking beans, greatly enhances the ease of digestion and increases overall vitamin content. Peanuts are not nuts; they are part of the legume family. Raw cashews can be toxic, as they must be boiled 30 minutes to remove the toxins; and are also not too politically correct.

**The healthiest nuts are: macadamia nuts, almonds, hazelnuts, filberts' nuts, walnuts, pecans, pine nuts, pumpkin seeds, and sunflower seeds.** These nuts and seeds are higher in monounsaturated healthy fats and are best eaten between meals as a healthy snack.

8.   POTATOES. Use: the red skinned potatoes, the dark brown-skinned Russet potatoes, the new purple potatoes, sweet potatoes,

or yams. **Sweet potatoes and yams are the healthiest potatoes to be eaten.** The white skinned potatoes are much lower in mineral content and have a much lower nutrient density value.

9.  DAIRY PRODUCTS. **Stay away from all drinking milks that come from cows and that have been homogenized from whole milk, to skim milk, to non-fat milk.** The drinking of milk today is very different from that of the drinking milk of many years ago. The homogenized process of milk destroys the molecular structure of the fat and protein molecule. This is the reason that fat and protein do not separate in today's milk. Milk is extremely mucus producing and very difficult to digest for many people. Some milk products such as nonfat yogurt, kefir, cottage cheese or low fat cheeses may be more easily tolerated. Milk and dairy products are best eaten with acid or sub-acid fruits, and most vegetables. **Certified raw dairy products**, where available, are preferable. **Coconut milk, almond or any nut milks are best as a substitute.**

10. BUTTER OR MARGARINE. **Use real butter**, salt free or slightly salted, and raw butter where available. Margarine is an artificially hardened or hydrogenated vegetable oil that is extremely difficult on the human system. It contains trans-fatty acids that have been shown to produce free radical damage. I think one of the best butters available today is *"Kerrygold"* from Ireland; they also make a wonderful raw cheddar cheese.

11. PROCESSED FOODS. Avoid eating highly processed, tampered or counterfeit foods like **salami, sausage, pepperoni, or baloney**. Also, canned or packaged foods with high amounts of: **preservatives, artificial sweeteners, bleached flours, hardened fats (such as margarine and shortenings), highly refined sugar products, foods that have been sprayed with growth hormones and antibiotics.** These foods contribute very little to our overall nutrient intake, as they are either very low in nutrient density value or very high in unnecessary or poisonous chemicals.

12. WHOLE FOODS. Eat whole foods whenever possible. They are much less likely to be processed and overeaten. **For example, eat the whole fruit as opposed to drinking fruit juice. Eat the whole grain,**

such as wild rice or 100% whole-wheat non-GMO, as opposed to processed grain, such as white rice or white breads or pastas.

13. RAW FOOD. **Eat a minimum of 50 to 70% raw food daily**. Raw foods contain many valuable enzymes and vitamins and other essential nutrients that can be destroyed in cooking. Make sure all raw food is cleaned properly to avoid unnecessary contaminants.

14. COOKED VEGETABLES. **Steam or slow cook your vegetables. Boiled vegetables lose all the nutrients in the water**, down the drain; save for soup stock. However steamed vegetables are not only more nutritious, they taste so much better. Fresh or quick frozen vegetables — vacuum-sealed — are best. Canned foods have lower nutrient density value.

15. SALAD GREENS. Use the dark green for your salads like **Spinach or Kale.** They are rich in **chlorophyll, the blood of the plant, a nutrient very healthy for the system.** Do not use the round head iceberg lettuce, which has a very low nutrient density value.

16. COOKED OILS. Avoid eating fried or highly sautéed foods at very high temperatures. A quick hot stir-fry is permissible. The high temperatures of frying adversely change the molecular structure of the healthy mono-saturated and polyunsaturated fatty acids. **Use either cold pressed virgin, or extra virgin oils, coconut oil, avocado oil** are best as they have the highest smoke point. The oils with the highest amount of mono-saturated fatty acids such as **olive or flax oil are best.** Standard oils such as **Wesson Oil, Mazola Oil, or Crisco Oil** are extracted with chemical solvent such as Hexane, similar to kerosene.

17. JUICES. **Dilute all juices that you buy in the store 25 to 50% with clean, healthy water.** Most juices, whether it is in a can, a bottle or a concentrate, even when marked no sugar added, **may contain added sugar.** A glass of juice **such as orange juice or apple juice is equivalent to the sugar content of three to five pieces of the whole fruit, minus the fiber.** Since we all need to consume more fiber, stick with the whole fruit — you get all the fiber and no sugar jolt. Juice produces a concentration of the sugar and acids that may be difficult for the body to handle at any one time.

18. DRINKING WATER. **Drink four to eight glasses of pure clean water every day.** Drink either **pure spring water, distilled, purified or filtered water.** You may purchase a home water distiller, a reverse osmosis filtration system, or a good solid carbon block water filtration system. Or a combination that fits on or under the sink. City water is a source of many pollutants and contaminants, which are hazardous to your health.

19. BLACK PEPPER. Black Pepper has volatile oils that are an irritant and very damaging to the system when heated. **Use the black pepper after you cook the food** or not at all. **Red or chili pepper is best,** being a stimulant to the system and not an irritant.

20. ARTIFICAL SWEETNERS. NutraSweet and Equal are artificial sweeteners made with methyl chloride and two amino acids, aspartic acid and phenylalanine. **Methyl chloride is nothing more than cleaning fluid**, the same fluid that your dry cleaner uses.

21. PRESERVATIVES. **Make an effort to use fresh whole foods, or quick frozen foods with little or no preservatives whenever possible.** Canned or packaged foods high in preservatives such as BHT or BHA are nothing more than embalming fluid.

22. WHITE SALT. Pure sodium chloride is harsh on the system and may contribute to hypertension. Use mineral salts like: **Real Salt, Himalayan salt, Celtic salt, or Kosher salt.** These are salts that are dehydrated seawater and have all the minerals from the ocean. **You may also use: kelp powder, *Spike,* or *Vegit* – these are seasoning salt mixtures.** Learn to use different herbal spices to enhance the flavor of your foods.

23. WHITE SUGAR. The over-consumption of white sugar will deplete minerals from the system. **Use Xylitol sugar, or raw honey, raw maple syrup, sorghum, molasses or the new pure raw sugar cane juice that has been dehydrated called *Sucanat*.** These sugars still contain some nutrient value. *Remember though, any sugar excess is harmful to the system.*

24. ALCOHOL. **Limit your alcohol intake to one or two glasses per day.** The over consumption of alcohol is the major cause of

liver damage as in cirrhosis, and is one of three ways that shorten American lives. Research has shown that drinking small amounts of alcohol may be beneficial to the system.

25. COOKING UTENSILS. **Use only stainless steel, glass, enamel, cast iron, Vision Ware or a reasonable facsimile for cooking**. Most aluminum pots and pans and utensils are extremely toxic and unstable, and can leak aluminum into the food. **Aluminum is thought to exacerbate Alzheimer's disease**.

26. CHEWING. **Chew your food**. Saliva contains many different enzymes necessary for the digestion of food to begin. **Mastication also breaks up the food to smaller pieces to allow for easier digestion. Monitor how many chews you perform with each mouthful.**

27. TOBACCO PRODUCTS. Research on tobacco products is abundant. The adverse effects have been well documented, and smoking tobacco is a major cause of deaths around the world. Need we say more?

28. SUPPLEMENTS. **It is impossible to get all the vitamins and mineral from the foods we eat today.** Taking vitamin and mineral supplements is the same as a good insurance policy. It is better to have slightly expensive urine than to be deficient in anything.

This is where a great product like **Prime Longevity** fills this important need for your body. **It is without question, the most potent formula on the market today. It is triple times the potency of its nearest competitor.** On the next page, we show the formula's table of ingredients that is quite amazing. Besides having greater amounts of nutrients, it also has tremendous amounts of enhancements (called **BioCore® Optimum**), to increase your **body's absorption of its vitamins, minerals, amino acids and enzymes. Don't be fooled – Prime Longevity is the most potent!!**

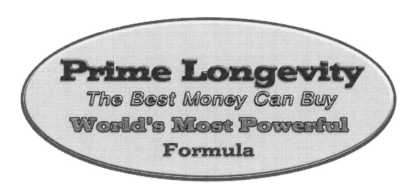

© 2017 Prime Longevity

## Supplement Facts

Serving Size 6 tablets • Servings Per Container 30

| Amount Per Serving | | %DV |
|---|---|---|
| Vitamin D3 | 2,000 IU | 500% |
| Riboflavin (vitamin B2) | 15 mg | 882% |
| Niacin (vitamin B-3) | 100 mg | 500% |
| Vitamin B6 (Pyridoxine HCl) | 20 mg | 1,000% |
| Folic Acid | 800 mcg | 200% |
| Vitamin B12 | 2,000 mcg | 16,666% |
| (Methylcobalamin) | | |
| Biotin | 500 mcg | 167% |
| Pantothenic Acid | 10 mg | 100% |
| (Calcium Pantothenate) | | |
| Selenium (krebs†) | 200 mcg | 286% |
| Chromium (Polynicotinate) | 500 mcg | 417% |
| Vanadium (Vanadyl sulfate) | 1,000 mg | * |
| RNA | 500 mg | * |
| Pomegranate | 275 mg | * |
| (fruit, standardized to 40% punicosides) | | |
| Acetyl L-Carnitine | 200 mg | * |
| PABA (para-Aminobenzoic Acid) | 200 mg | * |
| DMAE (Dimethylaminoethanol) | 200 mg | * |
| BioCore® Optimum | 150 mg | * |
| Amylase (from Aspergillus oryzae) | 5,250 DU | * |
| Protease (from A. oryzae) | 31,500 HUT | * |
| Protease (from A. oryzae) | 6,000 PC | * |
| Protease (from A. oryzae) | 3 AP | * |
| Glucoamylase (from Aspergillus niger) | 7.5 AGU | * |
| Protease (from A. niger) | 75 SAPU | * |
| Invertase | 600 SU | * |
| (from Saccharomyces cerevisiae) | | |
| Malt diastase (from Hordeum vulgare) | 2,250 DP | * |
| Lipase (from Candida rugosa, A. niger | 750 FIP | * |
| and Rhizopus oryzae) | | |

| Amount Per Serving | | %DV |
|---|---|---|
| L-Carnosine | 150 mg | * |
| CoQ10 | 100 mg | * |
| N-Acetyl L-Cysteine | 100 mg | * |
| Bamboo Extract | 100 mg | * |
| (*Bambusa vulgaris*, shoot ) | | |
| Giant Knotweed | 100 mg | * |
| (*Polygonum cuspidatum, root*) | | |
| Alpha Lipoic Acid | 100 mg | * |
| Glyconutrient Blend (milk) | 60 mg | * |
| (Containing galactose, fucose, xylose, glucose, | | |
| mannose, D-Glucosamine HCl, N- acetyl | | |
| Galactosamine, N-acetyl neuraminic acid.) | | |
| Green Tea Extract (leaf) | 50 mg | * |
| L-Glutathione | 50 mg | * |
| Standardized Boswellia extract | 50 mg | * |
| (standardized to 20% | | |
| boswellic acids, gum) | | |
| Standardized Tumeric Extract | 40 mg | * |
| (standardized to 95% | | |
| curcuminoids, rhizome) | | |
| Lecithin (from soy) | 40 mg | * |
| L-Cysteine | 25 mg | * |
| Cinnamon Bark Extract | 12 mg | * |
| (standardized to 2.25% Methylhydroxchalcone) | | |
| Inositol | 10 mg | * |
| 7-Keto™ | 5 mg | * |
| Boron (from Calcium fructoborate) | 1.5 mg | * |
| | | |
| *Daily Value not established. | | |

**There is nothing on the market today that can compare to Prime Longevity for both potency and its comprehensive formula**

## Order: (888) 486-2842

# CHAPTER 17

# LIVING IN OUR OWN SKIN

### Mirror, Mirror on the Wall, who is the fairest of them all?

Did you know that the appearance of the skin, healthy and glowing, or full of Facial Acne is one of the most traumatizing things a young girl or boy can experience? Looking in the mirror for a child **who has acne is proof of how bad skin makes them feel terrible about their looks.** Going on dates, or starting a new relationship, is hard enough as it is, yet throwing acne in the mix **can be terrifying or STRESS PRODUCING!**

Researchers at the University of California in San Francisco enlisted students who all had healthy skin. In a clinical study, it was found that **STRESS EFFECTS cause a diminishing in the skin's ability to function properly, heal wounds and fight diseases.**

These were all healthy vibrant kids. Imagine what stress can do to an adult's skin from: **a stock market crash, the loss of a baby, a pet, or a loved one, a divorce, war, bankruptcy, losing a limb, or a sudden illness.** By measuring stress levels of: **anger, confusion, anxiety, depression, fatigue and tension;** a **marked decrease in the blood supply to the surface of the skin was found**. This is what blocks the skin's ability to return to its normal function and glow.

Studies show after common stresses, meaning an average kid's college aggravation, **(tests, romance, growing up, etc.)** that a significant decrease was found in the skin's ability to breathe. **That means we are strangling and suffocating a child's skin with our stress problems.**

**Our skin is the only outside protection for our children.** It represents who they are to others. Are they a happy, healthy, and joyful person with a fulfilling stress-free life? What does your child show to the world?

Our skin cannot play poker; it shows what's in front of it. It cannot bluff – and pretty soon your child is **"Out."** And **the debt your child owes never comes back to their skin; yet healthy skin can respond positively.**

How is it possible, you ask?

Did you know **there is a direct link from a stressed individual's skin trauma to psoriasis, eczema, dermatitis,** and even to **premature aging**?

Dr. Mayora, clinical instructor in dermatology and cutaneous surgery at Miami's Miller School of Medicine says, *"In treatment of hundreds of patients over the years with skin conditions: (eczema, rosacea, acne, and psoriasis), I have seen how stress can aggravate the skin and trigger unexpected flare-ups, which create more stress for patients. Learning how to manage the effects of stress on your child's skin can help alleviate some of the anxiety and symptoms."*

So stop that right now! **Breathe, Relax, Look in that mirror** and choose a **Positive Affirmation. Say it aloud and mean it and by all means**; let that harmful stress go! Say it right now... *I love and appreciate my skin for always being soft and supple while covering and protecting my body!!*

**Fun Fact**

**Protein DNA Complexes,** known as **telomeres,** (the little cap covering the end of chromosomes) act as **generic timekeepers** and communicate with cells how long they will live. The longer the telomeres, the younger we are.

*Physiological Behavior* 2012 Apr 12; Vol. 106 No. 1 pp. 40–45

*"Long-term exposure to stress (and its physiological mediators), in particular cortisol, may lead to impaired telomere maintenance."*

*"Greater cortisol responses to the acute stressor were associated with shorter telomeres, as were higher overnight urinary-free cortisol levels and flatter daytime cortisol slopes. While robust physiological responses to acute stress serve important functions, the long-term consequences of frequent high stress reactivity may include accelerated telomere shortening."*

**"Being fearless doesn't mean living a life devoid of fear, but living a life in which our fears don't hold us back."**

**Dry Skin** is so annoying. Who hasn't peeled after a **sunburn** or flaked after a snowstorm?

Significantly dry skin can lead to **dermatitis**. That's a big, fancy word for an **inflammation** or **scaling of the skin**. The lack of proper: moisture levels, hydration, oxygen, and all those things our bodies long for, often create a rapid imbalance, and wreak havoc with your body's natural process of release.

Your body then builds up a barrier or wall preventing your skin from eliminating the cells in a healthy and a safe way. Often what we face instead is: dry, crusty, embarrassing and annoying **flakes, scales, and peels** that leave a messy trail behind.

**When someone is stressed, the level of the body's stress hormone (cortisol) rises.** This in turn causes an increase in oil production, which can lead to oily skin, acne and other related skin problems.

As dryness penetrates deeper, healthy *coenocytes,* which are **keratin-filled cells,** simply cannot reach the skin's surface. Imagine a miner underground just working away and there's an explosion and the mine caves in. The miner is trapped and can't get out. Your working cells get trapped and can't get out, impeding your ability to ward off drynesss, and all kinds of **environmental damage**.

Although the top layer of the skin on the hands and feet absorbs the most water, this type of exposure is followed by a rapid drying process called *Transepidermal Water Loss,* **(a type of water loss over which the body has little control),** that eventually leaves the skin drier. When washing dishes, etc, wearing latex-type gloves blocks the evaporation process and protects against the skin-wrinkling drying process.

In addition, many reasons why men and women lose their hair, Dr. Mayoral believes that **stress may be the primary reason for unexplained hair loss**. When someone is under stress, hair can go into the *telogen* (fall-out) phase. Telogen effluvium is a very common hair loss problem that can occur **up to three months after a stressful event.**

## With all those moisturizers on the market shouldn't we be flake free?

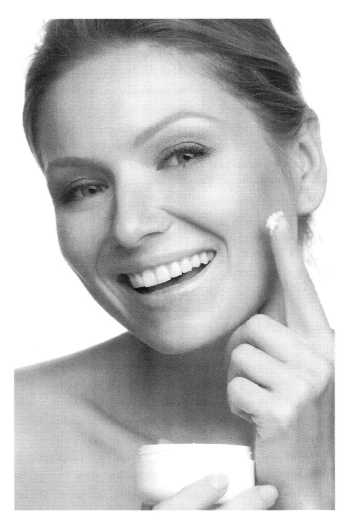

There are highly effective moisturizers out there and knowing what to look for can save you stress, time and money. Moisturizers that contain a healthy balance of **humectants** *(substances that promote the retention of moisture)* and **occlusives** *(protects the skin by sealing in healthy moisture and sealing out environmental bacteria)* are fantastic. Okay so what does that mean? **Glycerin is a highly effective form of humectants** and something as simple as a good **petroleum jelly is an occlusive. Hey, it works for babies and it can work for you!**

Humectants bind with water within the coenocytes, while **occlusives replace the lipids in the skins surface. This is important because it forms an actual physical barrier reducing water loss while sealing needed moisture into the cells.**

**Petroleum Jelly is also highly effective for healing and preventing chapped lips and elbows because Petroleum Jelly has been clinically proven to heal skin.**

UVA and UVB rays are dangerous and capable of inducing skin cancer. Strong sunburns increase your risk especially over a long period of time. Take 5 minutes, take 3 minutes, take 2 minutes; take 1 and protect your skin with a good and effective sunscreen.

Buy some cool sunglasses and use umbrellas and awnings. Wear a floppy hat and clothing that has UV protection like beach cover-ups, and enjoy the sun! However be smart and be safe. **Remember: sunbathing today creates skin wrinkles that show tomorrow.**

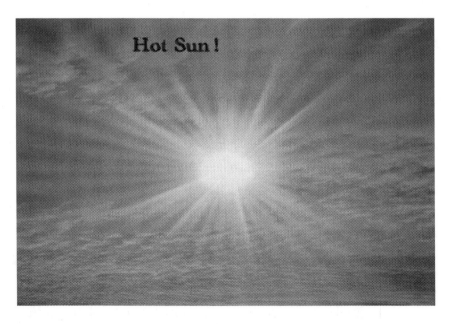

**Protection Tips**

Don't sunbathe or frequent tanning parlors.

Avoid exposure in the strongest sun (from 10 am – 3pm).

**Great skin and water fact to use to impress your friends:**

Why does the skin wrinkle after we take a bath or shower? The top layer of the skin absorbs water like a sponge when it is submerged into water. The more it is saturated with water, the more it expands and gets softer resulting in a prune-like condition we've all experienced.

Of course Nature has a good reason for this: **prune-fingers in water make grasping objects easier than flat finger**s – another survival mode essential to each of us.

Since fingertips and toe tips contain the thickest stratum **Corneum** (top layer of skin), this area shows **the most prune-like changes.**

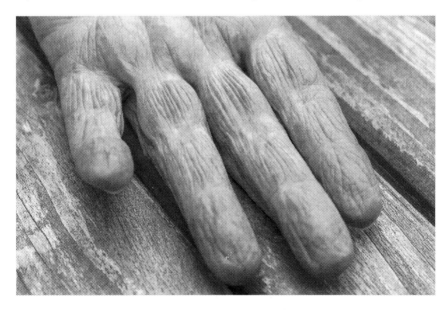

Although the top layer of skin on the hands and absorbs the most water, this type of exposure is followed by a rapid drying process called **Transepidermal Water Loss, which eventually leaves the skin dryer.**

Dry, scaly patches of eczema, etc, are an indication that the barrier function of the skin is not working properly. **Once the skin barrier has**

**been breached, irritants such as soaps and detergents can dry out the skin and cause deterioration of the already weakened barrier.** This causes eczema to become even worse. It also puts the skin at greater risk of exposure to food and inhalant allergens that penetrate the upper layers of the skin. **It's extremely important to repair the skin barrier with the use of emollients and wet wrap therapy.**

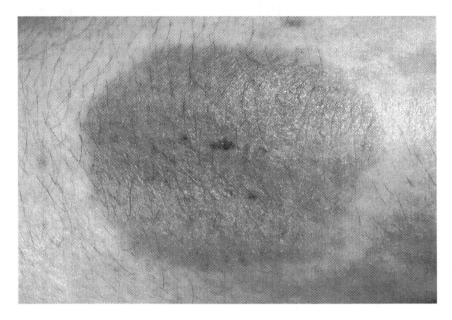

**Dry Flaking Skin**

**Dry Skin Helpful Hints**

- Limit Baths or Showers to 5 – 10 minutes. Use a shower water filter to remove the chlorine because it wrinkles the skin, and displaces the iodine in your body to wreak havoc on your thyroid.

- Avoid very hot showers or baths and use detergent-free soaps.

- Apply Moisturizer after drying off from a shower, or washing your hands.

- Use Bath Oils and Moisturizers daily. Thick moisturizers work best. **Avoid products with alcohol.**

- **Drink plenty of water throughout the day!**

**Additional Measures for Dry Skin**

**Lower the thermostat – Hot air is drier than cool air.** If you need to keep the room temperature warm, use a humidifier, it will put moisture back into the air.

**Drinking water is very helpful for your skin.** Drinking a sufficient amount of water is crucial to your skin because water aids in digestion, circulation, absorption and excretion. Since skin is made up of cells, each cell requires enough water for it to look healthy and vibrant.

The surprising fact about drinking water is that water will **reach all the other organs before it reaches the skin.** So make sure to drink enough, in order to supply extra water to your skin. This will not only show an improved difference in hydration, but it can prevent wrinkles as well.

*"Drinking water is also a cleanser – like washing out your insides. The water will cleanse your system, fill you up, decrease your caloric load and improve the function of all your tissues."* **– Kevin R. Stone**

**When cleaning, always use protective gloves to prevent damage to your hands.**

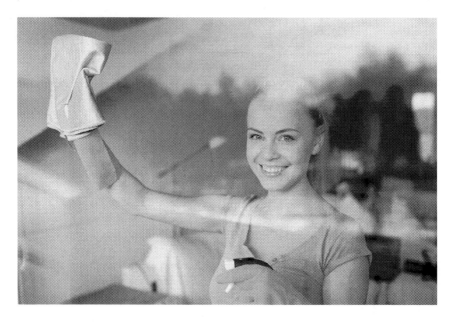

**Protect Your Skin**

**Time Tested Beauty Tips**

For attractive lips, speak words of kindness.

For lovely eyes, seek out the good in people.

For a slim figure, share your food with the hungry.

For beautiful hair, let a child run his or her fingers through it once a day.

For poise, walk with the knowledge you'll never walk alone.

People, even more than things, have to be: restored, renewed, revived, reclaimed, and redeemed. Never throw out anybody.

Remember, if you ever need a helping hand, you'll find one at the end of your arm.

As you grow older, you will discover that you have two hands; one for helping yourself, the other for helping others.

The beauty of a woman is not in the clothes she wears, the figure that she carries, or the way she combs her hair. The beauty of a woman must be seen from in her eyes, because that is the doorway to her heart, the place where love resides.

The beauty of a woman is not in a facial mole, but true beauty in a woman is reflected in her soul. It is the caring that she lovingly gives, the passion that she shows, and the beauty of a woman with passing years only grows!

**– Sam Levenson**

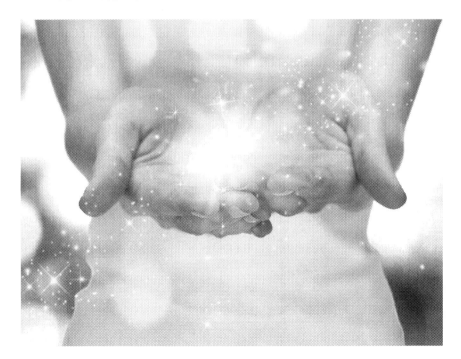

# CHAPTER 18

# CYCLES OF EMOTION

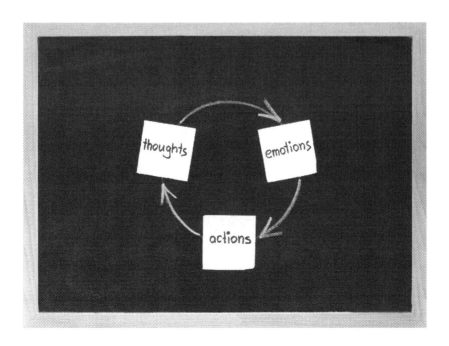

We would now like to explain *'the cycle of emotions,'* which occur in all of us. Understanding lessons of angers and resentments, as well as all negative emotions, is something we all desire. We want to put all negative emotions – not just anger or resentment – in a different light, the light of pure energy. We hope this narrative will allow you to change your perspective, to look to the lessons of life as **stepping-stones instead of stumbling blocks,** and to help you release your pain.

Let us first ask you a question, **"How does personal growth occur?"** Do we consciously move towards our own growth, or are we: kicked, battered, beaten, or traumatized into personal changes? Do any of you know of anyone that was born into a conscious family, where the parents taught their children how to express negative emotions in an uplifting, positive and growth-producing way? That seems almost funny, doesn't it?

Was there a picture book, or a video, or a movie? Or was there a game when you were children that taught you how to deal with: anger, fears, resentments, and depression, in such a way that produced growth without pain, fear, or hardship? **No!** Was there a time in your life when you thought those monsters under your closet were real? Was there a math test that you thought was the end of the world, or **how about losing your first love?** We know that it is possible to walk consciously to our own personal growth. We have been on the path; yet let us tell you, it takes tremendous intentionality and training. What happened when we were children? **How did we lose the magic, the faith, the trust, the belief and the fairytale? Where did it go?**

We learn as we fall and get up, that it is mostly through our pain and adversity that we grow. That will and that determination teach us how to strive to success.

Carrying Suitcases of items can get heavy over time. **Excess baggage always costs you something, just check in at the airline.** Sometimes carrying excess weight can affect our health and our heart. Other times from carrying: golf clubs, kids, handbags, etc. Eventually we become lopsided and uneven, and nagging pain kicks in for years. Allow us to give you a new way of relating to your past – and your emotional pain – that may help you get rid of all that excess baggage.

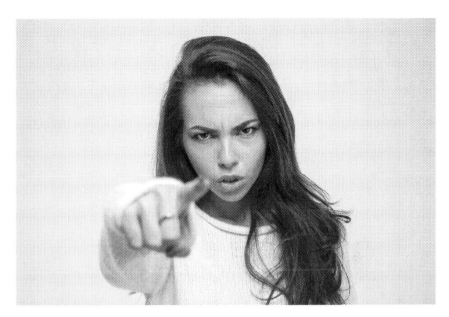

## Anger

**Anger** can be a double-edged power source. Physically, it is the most dangerous emotion for the heart and circulatory system. Mentally, it is the most intense, and fiery of all the emotions. Anger can generate the power for great actions being ignited by a legitimate grievance. **It can also cause you to lose all conscious and mental control ending up in pain for you, or someone you love.**

When it's bottled up inside, that intense fire can smolder away and produce the shattering pain of a **heart attack**, the devastating destruction of a **stroke** – or the eruption of an uncontrollable outburst that may engulf us and **burn a hole right through our stomach.**

**When we are the subject, or the target of a volatile temper, life has shown that there will be painful, and unforgettable long-lasting scars.**

As the subconscious rules, we tend to respond automatically. Just like when a doctor hits your knee with the rubber hammer. We react without thinking to an external force that jolted us from our peace, and the results will vary but they are rarely positive or enlightening.

Sometimes when we finally calm down, we regret our words or our actions that were spewed or hastened by our: tempers, discontentment, fear, insecurity, volatility, and frustration, **which we call anger** and we react.

Sometimes we regret having no response at all. How often have you said, *"if only I had said something?"*

Or how many times were we embarrassed for sticking our foot in our mouths? We get angry with ourselves, and we beat ourselves up, and the little voice inside us says:

***If only I had done something. If only I hadn't done something!***

We get angry! We get upset!

We rant! We rave!!

***And…*** we even give up!

When logically we knew, that if we had we been **thinking,** we would have expressed our emotion in a completely different way.

**Similarly without thinking, we get excited and enthusiastic about things and we end up with emotional pain, heartache and trauma;** which when we look back, **some reasoning and thought might have been helpful indeed! Pursuing things with a little less passion and gusto, and a little more thinking and reasoning could save us worlds of pain.**

**Have you ever felt that you cannot control, or direct your emotions?**

**Have you ever felt that you are at the mercy of unconscious forces,** sources or plans? The goal here is to gain understanding **and to be free**

to express our intensity of emotions in an appropriate, uplifting and a growth-producing way.

*There is always a lesson to be learned.*

We all express ourselves in different ways, with different emotions. Whether conscious or unconscious, the brain of every human being on the planet primarily works in one of **three ways: auditory** (our sense of hearing), **visual** (our sense of seeing), and **kinesthetic** (our physical sense of feeling).

**There is a cycle to all emotions.**

We relate to them either through our **mental** thought process (how we think), through our **emotions** (how we feel emotionally), or through our **physical** bodies (how we feel physically).

All three processes are different and separate. **How we think about things**, or **how we process information** on an intellectual basis, is very different than **how we feel about things** on an emotional level, or **what we feel physically** from our bodies relating to the physical world around us.

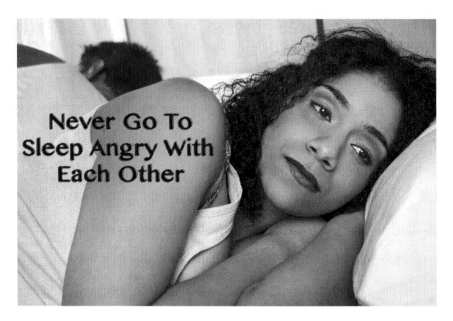

Never Go To Sleep Angry With Each Other

*Anger is always a secondary emotion directed outward,*
**where the primary emotion was pain.**

The emotional body, we believe, is the most misunderstood. So many of us on a spiritual path attempt to circumvent our experience on an emotional level. **We do this by thinking that we can (somehow), get rid of our negative emotions. However, our negative emotions are not within us on a physical level.** We experience our emotions physically through our bodies. Therefore, the emotions must express the same laws of physics that our physical bodies express. We can't change **what we feel.** We can only change **how we relate to what we feel.** Doesn't that make sense?

**These laws are expressed in the form of elements.**

**Emotions** come under the **water principal (constriction),** and are expressed through the body. Both **thinking and reasoning** come under the **fire principal (expansion),** expressed through the mind.

When the mind and body are in a state of balance, then the **air principal (neutral)** is expressed through our deepest truths.

Here then, is the cycle of emotions that each human must deal with, which come under the water principle and the 5 elements of the body. The first is grief, you move through your grief by looking to something that is greater than yourself, or you suppress it.

The highest emotion is grief, the element of Aether, expressed through the throat. **Grief is the loss of something – that feeling of emptiness when a loved one passes, or you lose something that was dear to you, or even when something you believed in, turns out to be a lie.** All cause a vacuum, which the law of physics says, *'the vacuum must draw something to fill it.'*

**Do you remember having that lump in your throat when you lost something? That lump always occurs with grieving**. You can accept the grief and move on with your life knowing that you are still a complete, spiritual being. On the other hand, you can suppress the grief and **start the downward cycle of the emotional yo-yo syndrome that all humans experience.**

When the grief is suppressed, we move down into the chest area, the **element of air.** We call this our seat of desire, and the law says, 'we must create something tangible to fill up that emptiness or void.

*A unique sigh may come from our chest. Have you ever been window shopping and seen something that you wanted, do you remember the sigh?*

**A man said to the Buddha, "I want Happiness."**
**Buddha said, first remove 'I', that's ego, then remove "want",**
**that's desire.**
**See now you are left with only Happiness."**

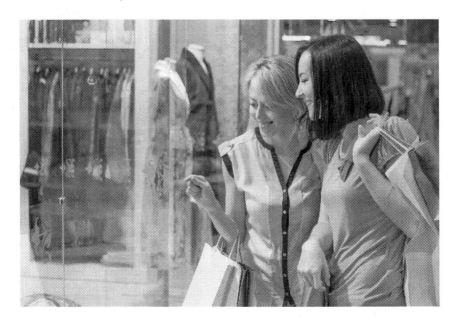

Once the desire is known, we drop down another element, that of fire. **Fire either produces the heat of energy to do work, or the heat that kills.** We either generate the energy to go out and work for our desire, or we feel the pain of not having our desire; that **then turns to frustration and then to anger of not having whatever that desire is.**

The anger either causes the fire of **heartburn** and **digestive problems,** or to the extreme – **the fiery, burning pain in your chest of a heart attack.**

*(Heart attack or myocardial infarction (def): When the blood supply to the heart is drastically reduced or completely shut off, causing the cardiac muscle to die from lack of oxygen. Over 1.1 million people experience a heart attack each year.)*

And the emotional result is that you either get the desire you crave, or you don't. Once you get it, you drop down to the next element of water.

**The element of water**, we call the seat of **attachments, or love**. Once we have the thing we desired (always something external), we now become attached to the very thing of our desire. Many people confuse attachments with love; the difference is – **love has no attachments!**

*When a partner or mate may say,* *"if you loved me, then you would* *do (xyz)."* *What they really mean is: if you want to stay attached to* *me, you better do...*

We have our desire. We love having it, *"Oh no, someone may take it* *away from me! I must protect it!"*

We now drop down another element to that of the **sacrum (lower back)** representing the element of earth **and the seat of fear or excitement –** the fear of losing whatever it is – which you just got attached to.

Have you ever become afraid of losing your attachments? Have you found yourself building up walls to protect the things you are attached to?

Maybe you've put locks on your doors, and added an alarm system, so that you would know whenever someone tried to take the object of desire away from you.

At some point through our own growth, we realize that **we are a** **complete person even without the object of our desire at hand.**

We realize that our attachment to our object has diminished and we can live without this item.

**What an epiphany!!** We now move upward and cycle back through each element with less of a charge or intensity about that desire.

**Earth**, the fear of not having the object of our desire has diminished.

**Water**, the attachment to the object is also diminished.

**Fire**, the pain, frustration and anger without the desire are also diminished.

**Air**, the object of our desire is now diminished.

**Aether**, we have returned back to grief and the vacuum. If it's not this object of my desire, than what is it?

**As we pass thru grief, we realize the desire is gone. We tell ourselves, "I don't need this anymore and, I am complete."**

Even though that experience is gone, somehow you experience that emptiness again and maybe even that loss again. You may ask yourself, *"If it's not whatever I just let go of – then what is it that I want?"* When you don't know, the process may start all over again and again.

Many feel the cycle is never-ending, just one desire after the next and we're always looking outside of ourselves, for that one something that will fill us up and help us to feel complete. The yo-yo cycle of emotions continues our entire lives, one desire after the next, always looking for something.

However, nothing external can ever fill that yearning and that void. We may understand that we are part of the vastness of the universe and that something greater on a deep energetic level is inside of us.

### *We call this 'Oneness.'*

**All emotions – both negative and positive – are either our stepping-stones or our stumbling blocks.** They produce the energy and pressure needed to produce the movement for our growth on a daily basis.

Each day you ask yourself, *"What might I accomplish today?"*

At the **end of each day,** ask yourself again, **"What have I accomplished today?"**

One never stays the same in life; you either go forward or backward, inward or outward, upward or downward.

**Yet, the lucky ones are those who feel a 'Oneness' with the great Universe.'** And whether they go forward or backward, they're living a path that is chosen by the Universe. So even going backward, they regard this occurrence as in their best interest.

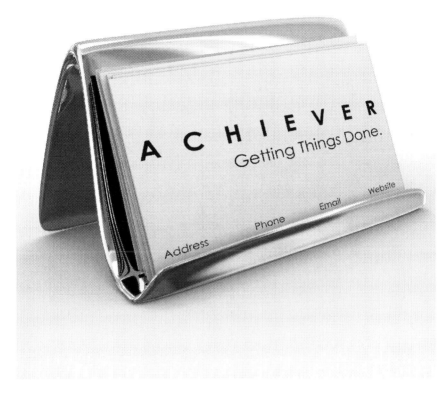

*Accomplish something each day!*

*"If we did all the things we were capable of,*

*we would literally astond oursleves."*

**Thomas Edision**

# CHAPTER 19

# 2-3 MINUTE TECHNIQUES TO DEAL WITH STRESS

You can use a number of methods to cope with stress, allow yourself to experiment to find the techniques that work best for you. We're giving you a smorgasbord of ideas and all of them work. Any avenue you choose will invariable improve your life. Some are fun, some are relaxing, some, take concentration, while others are effortless and quite seamless.

You've created your own scenario and story and now you can choose the technique that works just for you. **Like a kid in a toy store, play, have fun, try everything out and really enjoy the process**.

Here are some of our favorites:

**Muscle tension and release**: Lie down in a quiet room. Take a slow, deep breath. As you breathe in, tense a particular muscle or group of muscles. For example, you can squeeze your eyes shut, frown; clench your teeth. You can make a fist; or even stiffen your arms or your legs. Now hold your breath and keep your muscles tense for just a second or two. Then breathe out, release the tension, and let your body relax completely. Repeat the process with another muscle or muscle group.

You also can do a variation of this method, called "**progressive relaxation**." You start with the toes of one foot and, working upward, progressively tense and relax all the muscles of the one leg. Next, do the same with the other leg. Then tense and relax the rest of the muscle groups in your body, including your butt muscles, your stomach muscles and even those muscles in your scalp. Remember to hold your breath while tensing your muscles and to breathe out when releasing the tension. It's a great exercise!

**Rhythmic breathing**: We think that this process is the easiest and most effective because there's less mental work and more physical doing. Get into a comfortable position and relax all your muscles. When you want to keep your eyes open, focus on a distant object, when you want to close your eyes, imagine a peaceful scene, **or simply clear your mind and focus on your breathing.**

Breathe in and out slowly and comfortably through your nose. If you like, you can keep the rhythm steady by saying to yourself, *"In, one two – Out, one two."* **Feel yourself relax and go limp each time you breathe out.**

You can do this technique for just a few seconds, or for up to 10 minutes. You can end your rhythmic breathing by counting slowly and silently to three.

• Place one hand flat against your abdomen.

• Breathe in through your nose at a slow, even pace.

• **Feel your abdomen expand**, as opposed to your chest. You should **focus on the hand on your abdomen being pushed away from your body as you breathe in.**

• **The belly hand is the only one that rises on the inhalation.**

*Not only is this perhaps the easiest process – it also requires with the least amount of concentration, and delivers the most physically beneficial responses of lowering your heart rate, and blood pressure. As this occurs, your muscles will relax without one consciously thinking of it because slowing the breath, and lowering the heart rate are the most important factors in guiding the individual into a relaxed, alpha state.*

**Imagine a technique where you can control your body functions such as your heart rate, blood pressure, and your muscle tension.** Biofeedback does just that with a machine that will immediately sense when your body shows signs of tension, and it will let you know in some fashion by making a recognizable sound, or by flashing a light. This ingenious machine also gives you feedback when you relax your body. Eventually, you will be able to control your relaxation responses without even having to depend on the feedback from the machine. You can ask your doctor or your nurse to refer you to someone highly trained in biofeedback practices. *One side note is that **biofeedback can be costly.***

The people's choice, we are all blessed with a keen sense of imagination. As children we daydreamed, and as adults, we plan and visualize our success and our future. One of the most popular techniques known is "Imagery." **Imagery is a way of daydreaming that uses all your senses.** It is more efficient and effective when you relax and close your eyes. Close your eyes now, and imagine a Ferrari — is it red? Imagine a rainstorm, a fireplace or a clown. By closing your eyes, the vivid colors and pictures dance in your imagination and readily come to life. You begin by breathing slowly and feeling yourself relax **as you imagine a ball of healing energy, perhaps a white light energy, forming somewhere in your body.**

When you can *"see"* the ball of energy: **imagine that as you breathe in, you can blow the ball to any part of the body where you are feeling pain, tension, or discomfort. When you breathe out, picture the air moving the ball away from your body, taking with it any painful or uncomfortable feelings.** *(Be sure to breathe naturally; there's no need to blow.)* **Continue to picture the ball moving towards you, and away from you, each time you breathe in and out.** You may see the ball getting bigger and bigger, as it takes away more and more of your tension and discomfort. Once the tension, stress and discomfort have floated away, **'smile in your heart' and slowly count to three: breathe in deeply, gently open your eyes, and say to yourself, "I feel alert, alive and relaxed."**

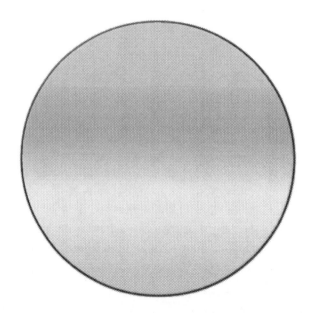

Okay, so at what point did you want your first car? Or that dress in the window? The cookie on the shelf, the cake in the window, the man or woman of your dreams: a vacation, a new refrigerator, a winning lottery ticket, a million dollars, a baby, a dream job or a college degree? What have you visualized in your life; **what have you created or made true?**

**Visualization** is a method that is similar to imagery. With visualization, you create an inner picture of: wholeness, wellness, happiness, contentment, and a wonderful, stress-free life.

**Hypnosis** with a professional, or **self-hypnosis,** is a highly effective technique for stress and pain relief. From the ability to stop smoking, to relinquishing, dealing with and banishing trauma; **hypnosis** is fabulous way to: release, let go of, and to deal with all forms of stress, or stress-related incidents, patterns and behaviors.

Hypnosis works by putting you in a trance-like state that is proven to help and reduce discomfort and all levels of anxiety. There are many qualified hypnotists out there, or you can learn how to hypnotize yourself. Whenever you are interested in learning more, ask your doctor or nurse to refer you to someone trained in this very effective technique. If you bring along a voice recorder, in just a few sessions, you may be able to duplicate the process on your own. **Before you select a therapist, find out if they are open to letting you record your sessions.** This is an important, money-saving process.

Look, over there!!!! **Distraction** can be used at any time to take your mind off your worries, troubles, stresses or discomforts. Distractions like: **watching TV, cooking, going to a movie, going to the gym, playing a sport, playing with your kids, comedy and comedy clubs, fixing something, cleaning, handy work, e-mails, listening to the radio, reading a book or magazine, traveling, getting out in nature, shopping, gardening, working with your hands, needlework, sewing, crotchet, playing with your pets, bathing your pets, or bathing your car, puzzles, picnics, amusement parks, building models, painting, or a variety of other activities,** will steer your mind away from the stresses or problems – and free your mind to a healthier and a happier life.

# AUTOGENIC TRAINING and BREATHING

When we think about any 2-3-minute techniques, we often question: can we relax, improve our stress levels, add oxygen to the body, and heal our own organs, and our hearts in just 2-3 minutes? **And the answer is, "YES."**

One popular and sure-fire way to relax is a fun technique known as **Autogenic Training.** Scientifically by far, it has shown the greatest results, in the fastest amount of time.

**Fun Fact**

Autogenic Training was developed by J. H. Schultz in 1912. The first of 6 volumes were published back in 1969 **with 2,600 scientific references!** Across the board: athletes, students, business people, and people everywhere, all improved with this simple technique.

> *Eighty percent of STRESS illnesses can be managed just with autogenic training!!*

So how can you use this tool to enhance your life and become Stress-Free? Easy.

Find a comfortable position – a reclining chair is ideal.

Now close your eyes.

As you breathe in, slowly say to yourself:

**"My arms and legs."**

As you breathe out say:

**"Are heavy and warm."**

Now imagine the sun beaming down onto your arms and your legs.

Do this for **three minutes daily,** for **one week.**

**Second week**, after the **3 minutes** with, *"My arms and legs are heavy and warm –*

As you breathe in, add the words:

**"My heartbeat is."**

As you breathe out, gently add the words:

**"Calm and regular."**

Continue on **for 3 minutes, while visualizing something calm and regular – like the pendulum of a clock.**

Continue daily for a week.

**Third week continue** the **2 earlier exercises.**

As you breathe in add,

"**My breathing is.**"

As you breathe out, quietly add, **"Free and Easy:"**

Visualize something you feel is free and easy. Often people imagine: **a bird gliding through the air, snow falling, the dew on the leaves, a running brook, a baby sleeping, a dolphin flipping thru the air** are all popular choices.

The fourth week continue your technique still for 3 minutes only; now you can **add three phrases that will bring you into your core, center, and light.**

As you breathe in focus and add:

**"My abdomen."**

As you breathe out feel safe and swaddled in love as you say,

**"Is warm."**

Soak in the warmth of the sun beaming down upon your abdomen.

**Relax and enjoy the process.**

As you practice, continue all 4 phrases – three minutes each, for one week.

As you've mastered the technique, **for the second month, be bold.**

As you breathe in **focus on your third eye, relax the tension around your eyes and furrows in your brow,** and simply say:

**"My forehead."**

As you breathe out, visualize being outside, warmly dressed, with a cool breeze blowing across your forehead – as you say:

**"Is cool."**

By the 6th week, you should be feeling great! Your body should be automatically relaxed and at peace. Now we can breathe in and add:

**"My mind."**

As you breathe out, know it, as you say it:

**"Is quiet and still."**

You can visualize a pleasant, quiet, still scene: **a park, a lake, a garden, a boat rocking gently on the shore, a plate of cookies, a glowing candle, a warm bath, the feeling of an embrace, your time in the womb, a bowl of fruit, cotton, a full moon night, glowing stars in the country sky, someone knitting, a book on a table, a library, or even a white scene of a snow blanketed area** – untouched, unscathed and just glowing in the light.

You have now learned how to relax your body, mind, spirit and soul in just 3 minutes a week. Remarkable and true, you are on your way to Stress-Free living and a better life.

*"During a panic attack, I remember that today is just today and that is all that it is. I take a deep breath in, and I realize that in this moment I am fine, and everything is okay."*

**— Max Greenfield**

*Life is too short to wake up with regrets.*

*So love the people who treat you right.*

*Forget about the ones who don't.*

*Believe everything happens for a reason.*

*When you get a chance, take it & if it changes your life, let it.*

*Nobody said life would be easy, they just promised,*

*"It would be worth it."*

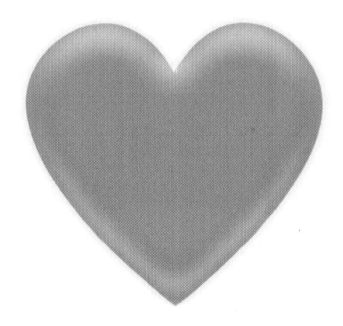

# CHAPTER 20

# SEX & RELATIONSHIPS

# It's not what I do, but the way I do it. It's not what I say, but the way I say it.

# – Mae West

### Lust and Attraction

With all judgments aside, **lust** is one the major reasons why we have survived as a species. Without lust (the sex drive), leading to reproduction, there would be no future generations of any species. Lust is defined as the craving for sex. And lust, by itself, has no further parameters than to complete a sexual act with another.

Lust and the **fulfillment of sexual desires** trigger a very potent biochemical response — the release of the hormones: **serotonin, oxytocin, dopamine and endogenous opioids** *(natural, opiate-like pain-pleasure chemicals similar to morphine)*. All of these substances together represent an amazing formula for **relaxing the nerves and muscles**, and **flooding the body with immense pleasure**.

Neurobiologists have detailed these bio-chemicals in their medical studies, to give you an idea of how immensely complicated the sexual attraction process is.

Over time, **lust evolved into attraction** — the difference being that attraction is a focusing of desire upon a specific individual.

While attraction can still be regarded as a **primitive, biologically based drive**, attraction is acknowledged to have a superior biological advantage to primitive lust, in that attraction motivated individuals to select preferred mating partners; thus safeguarding mating time and energy, and increasing the survival of the species.

Fortunately, humans do not identify each other as many animals do, which is by the sense of smell. People identify each other through **facial recognition, voice patterns, body language and an assortment of visual cues.**

Facial recognition is a lot more complicated than it sounds. A facial expression results from one or more motions or positions of the muscles of the face, which forms a complex language of non-verbal communication.

So literally, the actions of these muscles communicate the **direct thoughts and feelings** we are experiencing. Isn't that amazing!

Facial expressions are one of the primary forms of non-verbal communication that greatly influences attraction or repulsion between the sexes.

**Body language, gestures and eye contact** are the other major components of non-verbal communication, which tell volumes about our true motives and how we really feel.

In fact, one researcher, Albert Mehrabian, Professor Emeritus of Psychology, UCLA, developed his own *Mehrabian's rule.*

> **"When we speak to the opposite sex: 7% of meaning is in the words that are spoken, 38% of meaning is paralinguistic (the way that the words are said), and 55% of meaning is in facial expression"**

So clearly, our facial expressions and **voice intonations**, gestures, and other subtle visual cues *(the raising of the eyebrow, wink of the eye, a genuine smile),* are 93% of what the person perceives.

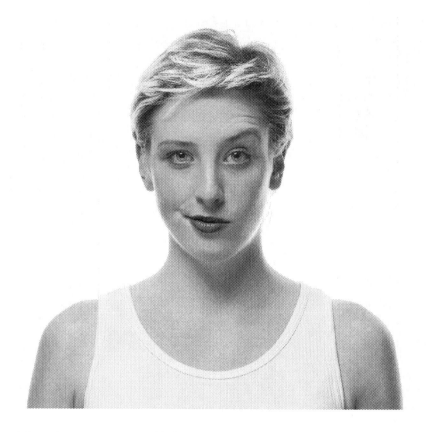

This phenomenon is called non-verbal communication. **And as stated before, 55% of what we reveal to the other person is done without words.** Researchers have carefully dissected and analyzed this process to an amazing science of its own.

Non-verbal communication includes: pitch, speed, tone and volume of voice, gestures and facial expressions, body posture, stance, and proximity to the listener, eye movements and contact, and dress and appearance. Think of it as everything that is visible, along with all that is heard.

And there is a specific name for a **genuine smile** that comes next. And once you learn this, you will never be deceived again!

## The Duchene Smile

And speaking of smiles, a French neurologist named Guillaume Duchene (who was crowned the father of electro-therapeutics), deduced that smiles that result from true happiness are the only ones that form a genuine smile.

**Duchene smiles** are formed by a unique, facial expression **by flexing the muscles near both ends of the mouth and around the eyes** – like the yellow smiley faces we've all come to love.

A Duchene smile contracts the zygomatic (fancy word for cheekbone muscles of the cheek and eye), forming **crow's feet**. The crow's feet indicate that the smile is **genuine** and that the person is **truly happy**.

How does this happen? There are several facial contractions that are involved:

1. The *Zygomatic* muscle lifts the corners of the mouth.

2. The *Orbicularis Oculi* muscles then raises both cheeks that form crow's feet around the eyes.

It is that **laughing smile,** which makes us smile back**. Smiling and laughter are great stress relievers**. The best medicine in the world is to laugh out loud. **And a smile can cure any heartbreak or wound, and touch you from across the room.**

### Elements of a Duchene Smile

A "natural smile" always includes:

➤ **Crow's Feet Around the Eyes** – *Orbicularis Oculi* muscles raise both cheeks

➤ **Raised Cheeks Smile** – *Zygomatic* muscle lifts the corners of the mouth

➤ **Remember 55% of what we communicate is in our facial expression**

## Duchene Smile

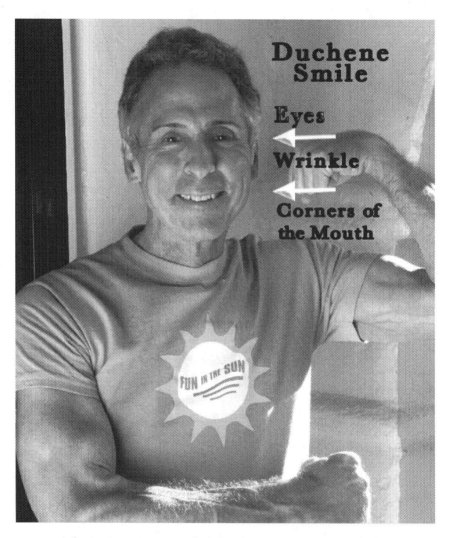

*The Zygomatic muscle lifts the corners of the mouth, while the Orbicularis Oculi muscles then raise both cheeks and form crow's feet around the eyes.*

### Fun Fact

Every form of facial expression has been analyzed by a researcher named Paul Ekman (who taught psychology at Princeton and Rutgers), and catalogued according to the anatomical muscles, eyebrows, etc., into the **Facial Action Coding System**.

**Did you know that neurologists have identified that facial attractiveness is processed to a large degree with the activation of the *left ventral tegmental* area of the brain?** What a task for our brain to drive us to happiness.

**Fun Fact**

**Being Single Used to Be More Detrimental to One's Health**

In the past, studies have often found that being single was far more detrimental to one's health than being in a relationship and living with a companion.

However, recent studies have shed light on the reality that **being in a bad or a negative relationship, or even running or hiding from conflict with one's partner, can be a powdered keg of trouble in a relationship and in your life.**

**Relationship Fighting — How to Survive**

**Troubled Relationships Are Dangerous**

The results showed that for those involved in troubled relationships, 34% were more likely to have heart attacks or other cardiac disorders, as opposed to those in positive relationships. Many scientists believe that stress from relationship problems is the culprit in the development of elevated levels of stress hormones and low-level inflammation of the arteries. That's a bigger problem than your mother or your friends saying, "I told you so"

**A Good Fight May Save Your Life**

Did you know that a good fight might literally save your life? **Studies have shown that couples who avoid confrontations and suppress their anger actually die faster, and in much greater numbers, than**

**those who push through and resolve their differences.** Agree now or disagree forever.

## Stunning Fact

In the study called **Marital Pair Anger Coping Types May Act as an Entity to Affect Mortality** (published in the *Journal of Family Communication*), lead researcher Ernest Harburg and his team followed 192 couples over 17 years. Categorized were couples where both members expressed their anger vs. those couples where the husband or the wife freely expressed their anger vs. a group where both partners suppressed their anger.

And the results turned out quite startling. **For those in the last group, where both partners suppressed their anger at each other when unfairly attacked, early death was double the rate as the other groups!** That's incredible!

## Suppressed Anger is a Known Killer

Out of the 192 pairs that were tracked, 13 of the 26 couples had the tragic rate of death where both members suppressed their anger during the study. **That's 50%!**

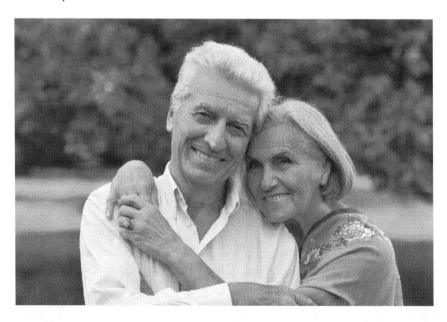

**Finding Solutions is the Key**

While the team of researchers was initially searching for information about heart disease, the lesson learned here is far more profound. First is this truth: **About resolving conflicts. A successful marriage cannot be achieved by those who are ignorant about resolving conflicts.**

Partners in a marriage have the privilege and unique opportunity to find solutions to their conflicts in a loving and respectful fashion and, to reconcile with each other.

Now we know that when one or both of the partners attempt to bury their anger, or silently brood over it, they will consciously or subconsciously resent their partner; and they will also do serious damage to their health and to their happiness.

Remember our earlier quote on anger: You will not be punished for your anger. You will be punished by your anger.

Whether it be brooding or resentfulness, or gloominess, they all are forms of anger – the proven killer of the heart.

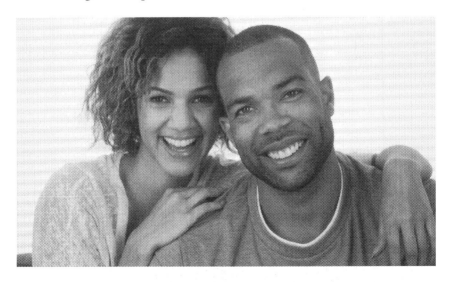

**ASPECTS OF A POSITIVE MARRIAGE**

**Focus on the positive aspects of your relationship.**

**Divide responsibilities in a way that satisfies both of you.**

**Acknowledge when you or your mate
changes, the relationship changes.**

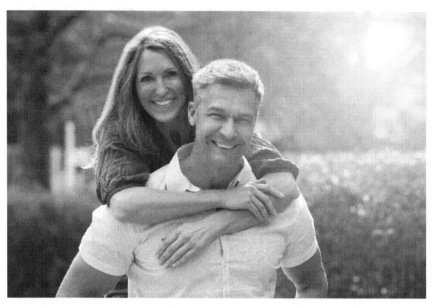

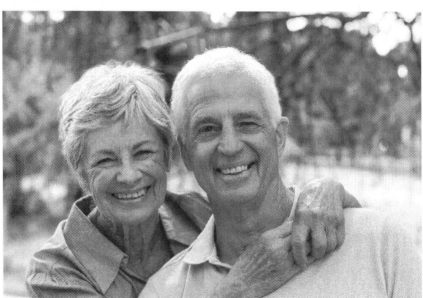

**Learn and know when it's important to compromise**

**Accept conflict, as a necessary element in**

**ALL relationships — Especially In a Marriage**

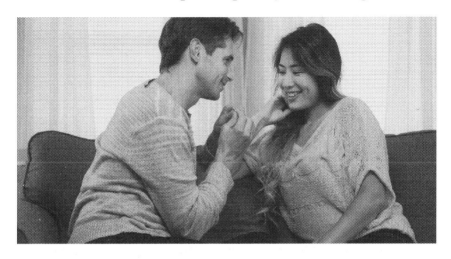

### Types of Attraction

### Women's Attraction to 'Bad Boys'

Why is the lure of **dangerous men** that attracts females, especially in their younger years?

Years of history from the height and craze of Rock n' roll showed us that teenage girls by the millions go "gaga" over: hard rock, electric guitars, banging drums, pierced punkers, rambunctious rappers, eccentric synthesizers, arrogant DJ's, crazed garage musicians and gangster music whose lyrical choices bash women, or tote sexual perversions in time with the beat. Why?

**Why does the traditional loner, noted outsider and anti-hero hero in movies, stir the passions of so many women? They represent mystery and excitement because they take risks; seem to have no fear, and exude a self-confidence that makes them appealing.**

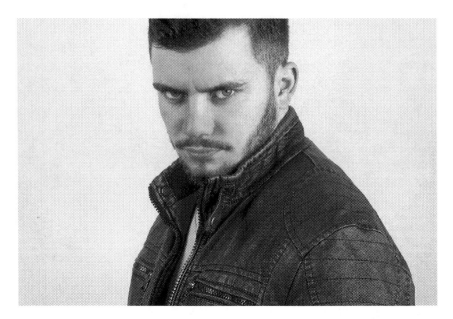

Ask a woman you know and respect about her attraction to James Bond, Sean Connery or other men or characters that play or portray villains, heroes, fighters, vindicators, maniacs or just play mean, despicable or outrageously narcissistic and fearless men — and she will swoon.

This phenomenon (the mystique of the tall, dark stranger) has been identified in psychology as the **Dark Triad** of personalities. Psychologists have identified these characteristics as possessing the combination of:

- **Machiavellianism (power focused)**

- **Subclinical narcissism (self-centered) and**

- **Subclinical psychopath (risk-taking, anti-social behavior)**

The lure of this to women has been undeniable.

### Still the Question, Why?

Testosterone is a hormone in men that is linked to the more dominant personality traits – outgoing personalities, charm, and excitement.

Narcissistic men tend to embellish their tales of sexual conquest, leading women to believe they are more sexually potent. Now there's a fun fact for you!

*The difference between Confidence and Arrogance is a thin line.*

*Confidence is believing yourself to be better today, than you were yesterday.*

*Arrogance is believing that you are better than others.*

**Women's Attraction to Males for Long-term Relationships**

While youthful girls are often smitten with exciting, dangerous boyfriends, these men are usually only successful in short-term relationships or causal affairs. Women, who are interested in a long-term relationship, are attracted to men who are altruistic. **Altruistic men were more attractive than handsome men. Adult women look for men who are reliable, responsible, productive and willing to build trust, intimacy and commitment to build a lifelong relationship.**

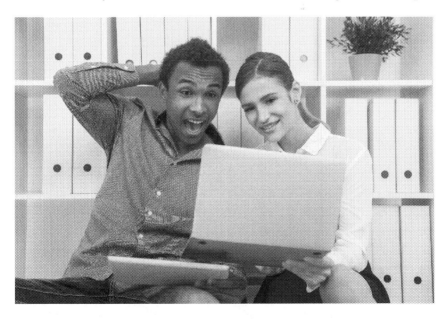

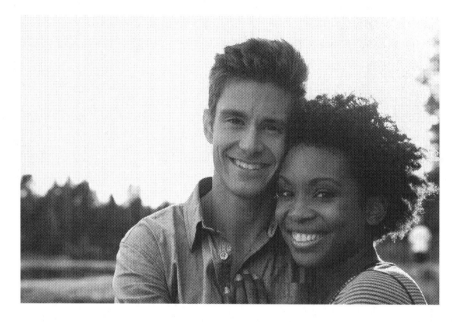

**Once a woman has found her mate or lifelong partner, the stress of looking, searching and even fielding through the bad boys of the past ends. Thus opening the floodgates for: tranquility, love, and a playground to share her sexual pleasure, intimacy, trust, and love.**

### Relationship Stress can shut down a Women's Connection to Others

When things are bad in personal relationships, women naturally withdraw from social interaction in its many forms. Many women become more closed off, often shortchanging their friends, co-workers and their loved ones.

In medical studies where hundreds of women were examined who had suffered acute coronary heart events (heart attacks, severe arrhythmias, strokes, etc.), doctors were profoundly moved because not only did they find the major physical damage directly related from relationship stress, they also found women withdrawing from social interaction to be consistent and quite alarming.

## Relationship Stress Equals Marital Stress

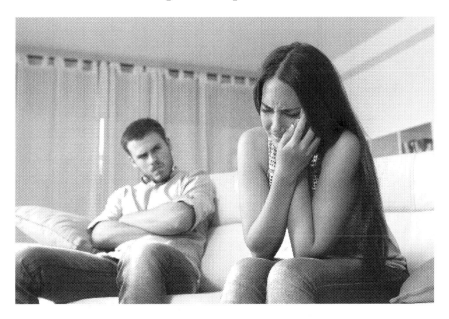

When we talk about relationship stress in research, we are talking about martial stress and its causes and effects. **Honestly whether the couple are married or not is irrelevant — relationship issues are always the same. If you're cohabitating with someone, this data applies to you!**

Relationship Stress has been linked with:

- Less social integration

- A lower sense of belonging

- Less tangible support

Since we are all beings with a strong and instinctual need of social connection, our mental and physical states hunger for that thread of connectivity, and to feel safe and to thrive in society, daily living and in our happiness.

## Can Positive Romantic Love Bring Us Benefits, Longevity and Happiness?

**YES**

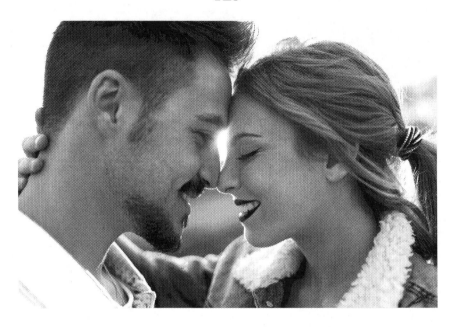

We now know that the feeling of Romantic Love with a partner deactivates or detonates a related set of regions in the brain that are connected to our negative emotions, and feelings of unhappiness. **Romantic love washes away doubt, judgment and fear, and creates and reinforces, our positive brain functions**. Maybe that's why they say, "**Love is the Bomb**."

Statistics show this is not a one-way street. Men have the same attachments and connections and the tug on one's health when feeling or being disconnected. **For men, it is an even higher statistic in damage, danger and permanent health problems.** So Men, if you are reading this, go out and fall in love!!!

Our longings, desires and frustrations with love often cause, "Yes" you are right — **they often cause stress**.

What's hidden in that romance novel that whisks a woman away, or what images are hidden and buried deep in the playboy magazine, or paraded vividly on the porn video that drive men wild? **What sex text, love letters or even advertisements set us off, or offers a thrill because the message or body before us turns us on in some dynamic fashion?**

We are drawn to sex: powerful, luscious, passionate, evocative, luring, titillating, accentuated movement, energy and physical desire.

Sex is natural, instinctual and downright fun. The onus we put on sex is the societal drive of the times. Countries around the world approach sex with different perspectives, views and modest lines. No matter what the upbringing, religion or background, sex has always brought pleasure, joy, happiness and life into this world.

The pent up tension and release not only relieves stress; it also opens the doors to stress-free living.

Everything we have taught you: from movement to breathing, from sound to satiation and appetite, and body image and gratitude, can be applied to sex. **Sexual pleasure, ecstasy and the release of orgasmic energy connect you not only to your lover or mate; but also to your own body, heart, spirit and soul.**

It is the recipe for life, with the whole meal, buffet and dessert laid out before our lives.

Yet why does it work? **In technical terms, an orgasm is the sudden release of built up sexual tension (climax) from the autonomic nervous system. The autonomic nervous system is composed of the sympathetic (controls stress response), and parasympathetic systems (controls relaxation of the body).** It sounds complicated and it's really quite remarkable.

The body has its own band of musicians and its own symphony just waiting to play your special and unique tune. Those **rhythmical contractions (undulation)** of the pelvic muscles create the number one hit song we call an **orgasm**. It's reigned on top of the charts for years!

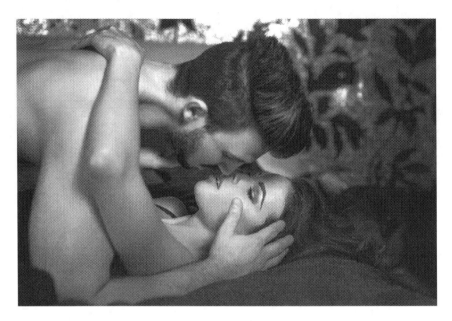

The other instruments or band members we'll call the **pc** or the ***pubococcygeus, anal sphincter, rectum and perineum.*** Together they make beautiful music. For women, we have a lead vocalist we'll call the uterus, and some backup singers, which account for the outer third of the vagina. Men have an electric guitar we'll call the ejaculatory ducts and bass player, trumpet and some drums, which are the muscles around the penis. Together they reach immense pleasure and a euphoric sensation, like the last stroke to the electric guitar that sends bolts of lightning through the crowd, reverberating your every cell; and we'll call that the climax. Followed by roaring thunderous applause, the band leaves the stage and the players head to their dressing room, and the body immediately packs up its instruments and goes into the state of **sheer satisfaction and deep relaxation.**

### The Emotional Response

Have you ever heard a song and it whisks your mind away? You may remember where you were the first time you heard that song and how the words made you laugh or cry. They may pump you up or bring you down — sex also can invoke an **emotional response.**

When two bodies, two hearts or two lives are intertwined, it can open *Pandora's Box* of **pleasure, aggression, submission and even emotional abandon**. Many people cry during sex, or after sex; the emotion is that strong. Many laugh, giggle and coo. **The doorway to our hearts opens, and deep emotions can be triggered, tapped into and birthed by two bodies joining in the dance of romance, passion, sex, lust and love**.

## Mental Response

Everybody's gone surfing: waves ripple and crash against the shores, foamy liquid gushes and flows, undulating and quivering, big waves, small waves, uncontrollable waves and little splashes of delight. Ebbing and flowing, pulling in and out, teasing us with their rhythmic power: beauty, magnificence and delight. Research has shown that our **brain wave activity,** much like those waves that soothe our soul and offer melodic harmony and the draw of the unknown, show marked changes during the buildup; climax, and relaxation stages of the orgasm. How could they not, when so much activity **roars with unyielding pleasure** and the joy of the journey? When we are set out to sea, we completely allow our brain waves to ride the surf of what we call **sexual pleasure and play.**

What an adventure! Back in the 1960's, **William Masters** and **Virginia Johnson,** both prominent sex researchers, published their studies on their sexual discoveries. They wrote in detail the **4 Stages of Sexual Response**. We'll call them breakfast, lunch, dinner and dessert.

**Excitement** wakes you up. This beginning phase can vary in duration from just mere minutes to several hours. It's kind of the difference between a pop tart for breakfast or a Sunday buffet. Physiologically, both include a quickened heart rate and an increase in muscle tension. **Blood flows and engorges the clitoris and vagina, and hardens the nipples, creating a full-body sexual blush. For men, the swelling of the genitalia results in an erection of the penis and a swelling of the testicles, contraction of the scrotal sac; and a secretion of lubricating liquid.** Many call it the love juice, which is a great starter for our banquet to begin.

For lunch, we'll look at the second phase—the Plateau. **The plateau is when the clitoris becomes erect. This matching of attunement creates what we've come to call the orgasmic platform.** This is a provocative and a secret place to launch from. It is a place to say hello before you're ready for the ride. Just as the horns toot and the bells whistle, this is this place where we gain more sexual activity, and the motions and emotions up the ante; and become even more intense. **This is the part people long for. It is this feeling and surge of excitement that we often wish could just go on forever.**

Then there's the dinner bell – **the Orgasm or the climax.** Our appetizers at this meal are physiological changes, and peaked intensity. **Our main course is served with a dish of an elevated heart rate racing with excitement, paired delectably with elevation of blood pressure. As our desire races wildly impacting every fiber of our being, then there's a buildup of semen just waiting to explode — coupled with delightful side dishes: our breathing increases and we salivate and pant like an excited puppy at the foot of the table, just licking our lips to be fed from the table of delight.** Then, of course, the *tour de force* main course – **the orgasm.**

Did you know that the orgasm is so powerful (and life-altering), that some individuals may even remain unconscious for a matter of seconds, or even for some minutes? To this the French coined the phrase *"petite mort"* or *(little death)*, **referring to the climax as a magical intoxication – and magical it is!** Whether second drifting to heaven, or the end of the concert as a sold-out success, sex does indeed relieve our tension; and it is a sure-fire way to release.

**Now the best part, even before the get go: the sugar sweet, delightful, fulfilling, marvelous treat and wonderland, the desert. We'll call this cream puff of delight the Resolution.** Just as the desert cart or desert tray is wheeled on out, we take a breath and lean back, pat our bellies and smile. **Here we enter an immediate sense of relaxation and utter bliss, sheer euphoria and sweeping satisfaction.**

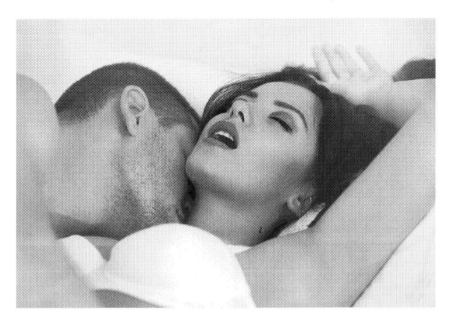

Our bodies return to normal, and there is a space that was created with joyous contentment: **wellbeing, and a deeper intimacy with our partners, and with ourselves. We relax, breathe easy and let go to a world that is Stress Free.**

**Love is an ice cream sundae, with all the marvelous coverings. Sex is the cherry on top. – Jimmy Dean**

**My wife wants sex in the back of the car and she wants me to drive. – Rodney Dangerfield**

**You only live once, but if you do it right, once is enough. – Mae West**

**An ounce of performance is worth pounds of promises. – Mae West**

**Too much of a good thing can be wonderful. – Mae West**

**When I'm good, I'm very good. But when I'm bad, I'm better! – Mae West**

## *A Prayer for the Stressed!*

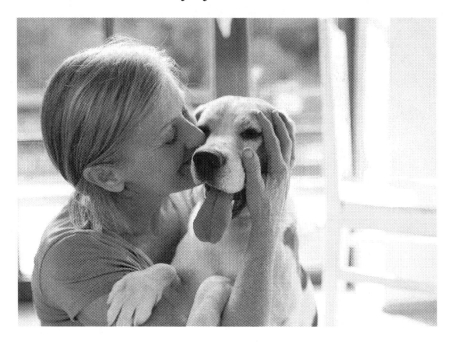

Grant me the serenity to accept the things I cannot
change, the courage to change the things I cannot accept,
and the wisdom to hide the bodies of those people I
had to kill today because they pissed me off.

Help me to always give 100% at work...

12% on Monday

23% on Tuesday

40% on Wednesday

20% on Thursday

5% on Fridays

And help me to remember...

When I'm having a really bad day, and it seems that people are trying to piss me off, that it takes 42 muscles to frown and only 4 muscles to extend my middle finger and tell them to bite me!

Amen

# CHAPTER 21

# ONE DEEP BREATH

As we close this story, we wanted to leave you with a most important secret. We wanted to share with you a solution to stress that can quickly change your life.

### Take 'ONE DEEP BREATH'

One Deep Breath can be accomplished easily, instantaneously, and at any time of the day. You can take one deep breath from any position – including standing, reclining, or sitting with ease.

It is the "Key" and infallible "Secret" to **Stress-Free Living through one moment in time.**

To Take One Deep Breath Simply Relax:

- Exhale completely and

- Empty your lungs as far as is comfortable for you.

You should already feel better. With just a little practice, you will be able to empty your lungs like never before. ***Make sure you're not forcing your breath***. Now that you're stress-free, **everything needs to be an effortless flow.**

- As you're relaxing, gently inhale as much air as you can.

- While your lungs are full, pause your breathing for five seconds of time, and then gently exhale.

**You can use this technique at anytime, as 4 to 7 seconds will work beautifully.**

- When you're ready to exhale, gently let go. There's no need to push, or to rush the exhale. **Give yourself the time and enjoy the process.**

### Doesn't this feel wonderful?

- You can even add a sound and let the air release with a glorious Sigh.

- Let the relaxing feeling ripple down your body: relaxing your hands, feet, legs, neck, shoulders and even your mind.

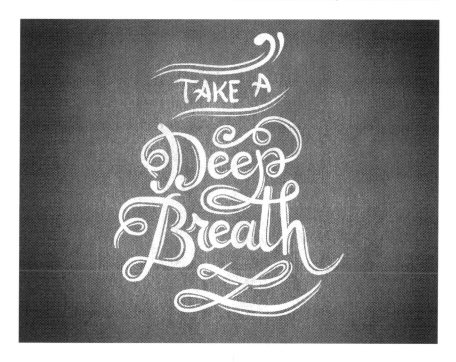

### When to Use One Deep Breath

Use this anytime you feel stressed, because something inside you was smart enough to know you are capable of relieving stress from your life. Something told you to pick up this book and to learn the tools, techniques and secrets to a healthier, happier and stress-free life.

And the beauty of this technique is that by simply following the instructions, **your body will respond positively whether you believe in the process or not.** This is because the body naturally follows the mind. Just like when you fell threatened, your mind signals your body to go into the *fight-or-flight response.*

This process is the absolute reverse. When you deep breath, your mind triggers your body to slow down into an **alpha state** (a natural state of relaxation). Every night, right before we go to sleep, our bodies quietly drift into an alpha state.

## One Deep Breath

Is useful anytime you'd like to slowdown your thoughts, or anytime you desire to tune into your Higher Self. All of this can be achieved and accomplished with 'One Deep Breath.' In addition to relieving stress and expanding your awareness, performing deep breaths benefits your entire being by bringing in more oxygen, which is 'food' for all the cells in your body.

## The Benefits of One Deep Breath

- Manage your stress

- Reduce the effects of your stress

- Balance your emotions

- Immediately calming your nerves

- Gently quieting your mind

- Finding inner peace

- Laser Sharp Focus

- Improve your mental function

- Tune into your Higher Self

- Release the tension in your mind, body and soul

- A Healthier and Happier Life

## A String of Pearls

By linking one deep breath after another, you will create a pathway that will lead to the ultimate treasure, the happiness of your life.

Imagine if you could manage your stress not just for: a second, or minutes, or hours, or even for a day; imagine a life of Stress Free Living!

**Just one deep breath** can help you manage your stress for a several minutes.

**Just five minutes of deep breathing** can help you manage your stress for over an hour.

**Just fifteen to twenty minutes of deep breathing** can help you **manage your stress for several hours.**

Imagine the increased joy in your life, and the ultimate benefits by simply taking one deep breath after another.

**The World Is Yours**

We've enjoyed being on this journey with you. Now is the time to celebrate and relax, and enjoy the Life that is meant to be yours.

Pass this book on. Help someone you care about and love. Or just read it and reread it, and each time you dive in, gift yourself with a moment of deep breathing, deep joy and deep happiness.

All of these tools work. Find the one that resonates and works best for you.

Do your friends a favor, and let them know how this book has helped you begin a whole, new chapter in your life by integrating these powerful techniques.

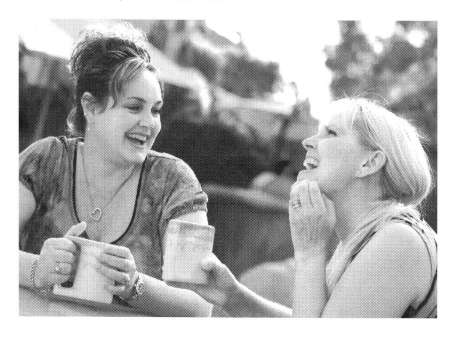

**Be kind to yourself.**

**You are amazing!**

To Your Happiness,

Dr. Eliezer Ben-Joseph

Richard Lewis, M.A.

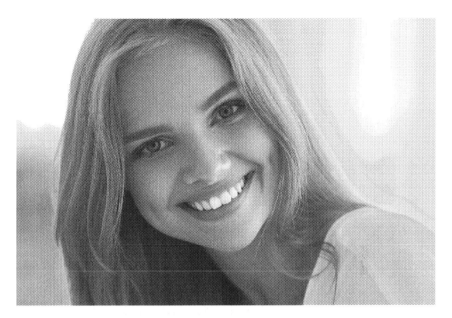

### Recipe for Happiness

2 Heaping cups of patience

1 Heart full of love

2 Hands full of generosity

1 Dash of laughter

1 Head full of understanding.

Sprinkle generously with kindness

Add plenty of faith and mix well.

Spread over a period of a lifetime

and share with every friend you love.

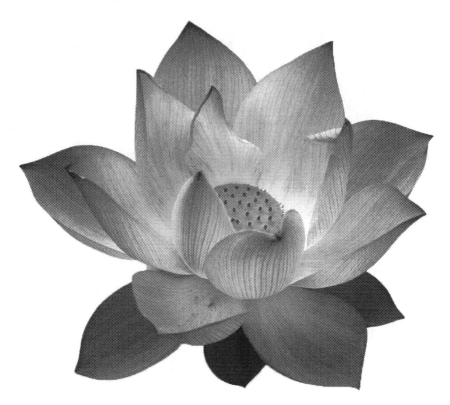

Disclaimer: All of these exercises have been proven to work effectively in Stress Free Living. Professional Guidance is always the best care. If you are unsure of an exercise wait, ask, seek coaching or ask your physician. Do not try all these exercises by yourself, unless you are clear on their safety and connection to your own wellness, health and success.

We are here for you as a resource, guide, and library to your wellness journey. We are happy to guide you to the safest, most effective tools designed just for you!

To Your Health!

Dr. Eliezer Ben Joseph

Richard Lewis, M.A.

Our website: smyfwd.com

## Dr. Eliezer Ben Joseph

Dr. Eliezer Ben-Joseph's research has pioneered the industry of health-related natural science.

With over 30 years of experience as a naturopathic physician, Dr. Eliezer Ben-Joseph has seen the destructive, unhealthy changes in our society due to a lack of proper diet, exercise and prevention of disease. Wanting to make a change towards wellness for the world, Dr. Eliezer Ben-Joseph researched modalities to revitalize and regenerate our bodies at the deepest cellular levels.

His first product, **Prime Longevity**, is a benchmark product tapping into every aspect of our physiology and its utmost potential. Briefly, Prime Longevity is the **most potent formula of vitamins, minerals, amino acids, and herbal extracts** on the market today.

Dr. Eliezer Ben-Joseph has a vast list of credentials that have taken him around the world. He has been knighted in the prestigious **"Hospitaller Order of Saint Lazarus of Jerusalem,"** and was conferred as **the "Grand Commandeer' of the Order"** – receiving the designation of **"Knight of Honor Cultural attaché.'"**

He has also been knighted in the **'Sacred Medical Order of the Knights of Hope,** and was appointed as the **'Grand Naturopathic Physician'** of the Order, and awarded the grand honor of *'Order pro Merito Spes.'* The main purpose of these long-standing, charitable organizations is to **administer medicine to heal the poor** in hospitals that the **Knights of Hope** have built around the world. This type of free medical services is referred to as **Monastic Medicine**.

Dr. Ben-Joseph is a board certified traditional naturopath (from Clayton College of Natural Medicine) with a full practice residing in El Paso, Texas.

He holds degrees **of MD (MA) Medicina Alternativa and a D.Sc. (Doctor of science)** from the **'Open International University for Complementary Medicines'** in Sri Lanka.

He has received both a **BS and MS in science** while studying **Chiropractic and Osteopathic medicine** in Israel.

Dr. Ben-Joseph studied Ayurvedic Medicine in a temple in India, and Physical Therapy in Amsterdam, where he received a **'Doctor of Philosophy in Hospitaller Medicine'** [*Honoric Causa*] from the **'PanAmerican University of Natural Medic**ine.'

He has studied herbology and 'Indigenous American Native Spirituality' and is a proud member of the **Oklevueha Native American Church**.

Dr. Ben-Joseph is also a **master herbalist, iridologist, certified RAYID Master** (psychological assessment of the iris of the eye), and an instructor in **Polarity Therapy and therapeutic bodywork**.

He is also **a certified personal trainer, a holistic health instructor, and has taught diet, nutrition, therapeutic bodywork, and personal development for over 25 years.**

Dr. Ben-Joseph was the **founding President of the Texas Naturopathic Medical Association,** served on the **Board of Directors of the American Naturopathic Medical Association**, and served as **Science editor of the Journal of the American Medical Association.**

He also sat on the **Board of Governors of Capital University** in Washington D.C.

Quite involved in community service in El Paso, Dr. Ben-Joseph has served on the **Board of Directors of the Shelter for Battered Women for over 17 years** and has served on the **Nutrition and Health Commission of the Paso Del Norte Health Foundation for the city of El Paso.**

Dr. Ben-Joseph is also the host of the top-rated **"Natural Solutions Radio,"** a call-in talk-radio show **on KTSM 690 Talk Radio** in El Paso, Texas **for the past 18 years**.

**Dr Ben-Joseph owns and operates one of the largest comprehensive, naturopathic outpatient facilities in the United States.** Dr. Ben-Joseph has **designed and implemented holistic protocols for the treatment of AIDS, cancer, and other degenerative diseases worldwide.**

## Richard Lewis, M.A.

After receiving a B.A. in Psychology through study at George Washington University, Emerson College and New York University, Richard Lewis earned a Master's Degree in Humanistic Psychology from Ryokan College in Los Angeles. Throughout his twenties, he was trained in a variety of holistic healing techniques: Acupressure, Reflexology, Swedish massage, Shiatsu, Deep Tissue Manipulation and Rolfing.

In addition to holistic physiotherapy, he also combined breathing relaxation, corrective-stretching and stress management techniques to help clients reduce stress and enhance their personal and/or professional performance. It was in the 1970s, that Lewis met Dr. Ben-Joseph who impressed him with his incredible background in almost every holistic method.

To assist his patients ever further, Lewis realized that his clients needed to be following an effective, therapeutic method of working the painful muscles gently; so as to utilize healing movements for the days that the clients were on their own. Over time, he became an expert in corrective stretching techniques tailored to each patient's needs.

Over his 35 years of therapy practice, Lewis developed his *"Stress-Relief Stretching"* for: relaxing physical and emotional tension, for "turning off" the body's cortisol stress response, for reducing cardiac exertion, for calming the nerves and clearing the mind.

Planning for a second career after physiotherapy, Lewis trained extensively in Photoshop Computer Graphics for the last 12 years.

His collaboration with Dr. Ben-Joseph is the culmination of thirty-five-years experience in the metabolic connection between stress, cortisol, and body fat; offering the reader insights to help achieve the body they desire, **along with a myriad of tools for stress management and a happier life.**

*Please enjoy this excerpt from my latest book on Diet and Nutrition.*

## Missing My Life

By Dr. Eliezer Ben-Joseph

When I was in first grade, I ran my first experiment. It was a nutrition experiment and I was the subject. Looking back it seems rather funny this little kid with a big, expansive mind looking for solutions. It's a twist of fate in the memory. Imagine that's who I was.

Some things never change.

I noticed that often I would fall asleep at my desk. Now most people would think I just had a boring teacher, which was probably true and I hope she's not reading this book right now. However, the truth is, I just didn't feel great. I felt sluggish and tired. My mind would wander a million miles away, and I just couldn't focus on the lesson at hand. Not to mention that I got hit with the ruler on the back of my head for not paying attention. So that alone, is a reason to wake up, yet somehow my body just didn't want to comply. Then on other days, I felt great – my energy was abounding. I was funny and pretty smart, kind of sharp, and incredibly personable; and on those days, I couldn't figure out why all my days weren't like that. No bruises on the side of my head from the teacher and pretty darn good days to be a kid.

What was different?

I decided to do an experiment with my breakfasts. If I ate one thing, how did I feel? Could I pass my math test if I ate one food or one fruit or one grain that was different than yesterday? Did pancakes affect me like waffles or toast or hot cereal or eggs or juice or…

I was a living experiment and what I found was crazy. I could actually navigate my day by what I ate. In first grade, I had figured this out.

I have since been on a lifelong journey to know why, and to learn the truth.

It's so confusing: eat this; don't eat this. Milk is good for you; milk is bad for you. Oil is good for you; oil is bad for you. Wine is good; wine is bad... Who and what do we believe?

Book after book tells us one thing or the other: this fad, this diet, this collection of what to do, and what not to do, could drive a person mad.

Grab all of your food books, diet books, nutrition books and latest fads and throw them all away. Cut up the pictures, make collages, or wallpaper your kitchen with the milk or fruit photos. Use them as kindling: bind them together to make cute tooth brush stools for your small children, line bird cages, make origami art, press flowers between the pages, just stop reading them and driving yourself insane.

I will teach you the truth about nutrition. You don't need to be sick, or tired or unhappy with your body ever again. Today you are on the pathway to your optimal health. This book is the gateway and the door to your health for your magnificent life.

I have dedicated my life to giving you the answers. To uncovering the truths and to figure out a way to share it, where you can: enjoy it, relish it, live it, and have fun with it. This book is a gift from myself, and my partner, to you.

From my 1<sup>st</sup> grade Self, let's start with breakfast!

Printed in the United States
By Bookmasters